ADJUST
YOUR BRAIN

A Practical Theory
for Maximizing Mental Health

Paul J. Fitzgerald, Ph.D.

BOOKS

Winchester, UK
Washington, USA

ADJUST
YOUR BRAIN

A Practical Theory
for Maximizing Mental Health

Paul J. Fitzgerald, Ph.D.

First published by O Books, 2007
O Books is an imprint of John Hunt Publishing Ltd.,
The Bothy, Deershot Lodge, Park Lane, Ropley, Hants, SO24 0BE, UK
office1@o-books.net
www.o-books.net

Distribution in:

UK and Europe
Orca Book Services
orders@orcabookservices.co.uk
Tel: 01202 665432 Fax: 01202 666219 Int. code (44)

USA and Canada
NBN
custserv@nbnbooks.com
Tel: 1 800 462 6420 Fax: 1 800 338 4550

Australia and New Zealand
Brumby Books
sales@brumbybooks.com.au
Tel: 61 3 9761 5535 Fax: 61 3 9761 7095

Far East (offices in Singapore, Thailand, Hong Kong, Taiwan)
Pansing Distribution Pte Ltd
kemal@pansing.com
Tel: 65 6319 9939 Fax: 65 6462 5761

South Africa
Alternative Books
altbook@peterhyde.co.za
Tel: 021 447 5300 Fax: 021 447 1430

Text copyright Paul Fitzgerald 2007

Design: Stuart Davies

ISBN: 978 1 84694 055 2

A CIP catalogue record for this book is available from the British Library.

Printed in the US by Maple Vail

Dr. Fitzgerald's book offers a clear and in-depth understanding and explanation of mental illness from the perspective of both patient and scientist. Dr. Fitzgerald wonderfully presents his personal exploration of his scientific and subjective experiences with mental illness.

Dr. Michael Heitt, Ph.D., Assistant Professor, Department of Psychiatry and Behavioral Sciences, Johns Hopkins University

Paul Fitzgerald has written a concise and easy to read book on the use of drugs to treat mental illness. His thesis is that most patients could benefit from a carefully selected combination of drugs that target several different chemical systems in the brain. Regardless of whether he's right, the book is informative about how brain chemistry works.

Dr. Joseph LeDoux, Ph.D., University Professor
New York University, author of *The Emotional Brain* and *Synaptic Self*

In this book, Dr. Fitzgerald proposes nothing less than a Unified Theory of human affect, personality, and motivation based on the balance of neurotransmitter systems in the brain. Furthermore, he argues that achieving neurotransmitter balance is essential for living life to its full potential. This is an elegant and provocative idea shaped equally by academic research and by personal experience. The author's own struggle with depression has granted him a unique perspective and a sense of urgency to comment on the promise of psychopharmacology. Dr. Fitzgerald advocates a deeply humanistic view, in which suffering is not an inescapable consequence of the human condition. He also convincingly argues that this is not a utopian goal, but within reach of modern medicine. Although the book never strays from arguments grounded on current research, it provides a condensed primer on brain function and it is written in an accessible manner that makes it equally enjoyable to all readers. It makes fascinating reading both for the wealth of information it provides and for its deep social and philosophical implications.

Dr. Christos Constantinidis, Ph.D., Assistant Professor, Department of Neurobiology & Anatomy, Wake Forest University School of Medicine

ACKNOWLEDGEMENTS

I'd like to first thank my family and various doctors for nursing me back to health from a state of severe depression five years ago. Without their tremendous support, I would not have been around to write this book.

Next I'd like to thank my agent, Sally van Haitsma of the Castiglia Literary Agency, for believing in the book when almost no one else did. Sally also provided invaluable editing of the manuscript.

I'd also like to thank my colleagues and mentors at Johns Hopkins and various other universities for giving me feedback on earlier versions of the manuscript. Their input led to a much better final product.

I'd like to finally extend thanks to John Hunt at O Books for taking on this somewhat unusual project. He saw potential where other publishers were afraid of the controversy that might follow.

www.brain-drugs.com

CONTENTS

INTRODUCTION

General Considerations

As with any new and provocative theory, this book is a work in progress, and some of the ideas presented are sure to change over time as research scientists like myself delve deeper into the brain, applying tools and methods not yet devised. I believe it nonetheless represents a significant and perhaps massive step forward for the field of psychiatry, both in a theoretical and a practical sense. In attempting to understand general principles of brain function that characterize different types of mental illness, including my own bipolar illness, I may have not only stumbled upon important principles for treating these illnesses but also uncovered basic brain characteristics that drastically affect our experience of the world. I have a Ph.D. in neuroscience from Johns Hopkins University, I am currently performing brain mapping studies at the Krieger Mind/Brain Institute of Johns Hopkins, and in my free time I have done extensive research on mental illness and the effects of psychiatric drugs.

The field of drug-based, biological psychiatry—the focus of this book—is really still in its infancy, as most of the commonly used drugs are no more than fifty years old, and even Prozac is less than twenty years old. Therefore, it is not surprising that there is a good deal of disagreement regarding which drug regimen—including even which class of drugs—to use on a given mentally ill individual. Moreover, many people with overt mental illnesses, even when given what are thought to be the best drugs, are not able to function normally and remain occupationally impaired even after years of tinkering with their drugs and dosages. However, some people do get dramatically better with drug treatment—psychiatrist Peter Kramer has argued that some people can even be made 'better than well' by Prozac, for example—and I am living proof that other drugs can also make one better than well (see Chapter 2). The existing pharmaceutical drugs are very powerful and potentially extremely effective *when used properly*, though in the field of psychiatry today there is no such consensus on how to use these drugs. Moreover, some of the more widely believed tenets of the field, such as that the most effective drugs for treating schizophrenia are the antipsychotics, may simply be wrong. So because of all this confusion, I have written this book in an effort to provide a coherent, unified framework for understanding the various mental illnesses, with the hope that such a framework will lead to much more effective drug treatment and higher quality of life for a large number of people. Indeed, this is a very exciting time for psychiatry, as it may now come much closer to reaching its full potential, with very positive consequences for society and humanity in general.

Actually, I like to think this is more than just a book about psychiatric drug treatment of the mentally ill. It also has at least two other major points of interest: one is that it provides a greater description of how the brain works and what it means to experience the world as a human being, and the other is that it indicates that psychiatry is no longer just of interest to very sick persons but also may help many so-called normal people have a much better life and live up to their full potential. Regarding the first point: I think people tend to think that others experience the world in a very similar manner to themselves, and perhaps that minor differences in temperament and major differences in life history explain the diversity of human behavior. I think my book explains that this is not the case. On the second point: The Adjustment theory, which involves adjusting two or three brain neurotransmitter systems in a particular way with drugs, should make life better both for the mentally ill and also for perhaps nearly everyone else. And if The Adjustment is very potent with the existing pharmaceutical drugs, and we pursue such treatment on an international scale, then the world may indeed become a much better place, partly because both human behavior and society might change to make it such a place. So we may be living at a very exciting time!

Nuts and Bolts of a Theory

Any theory reflects the biases and limited knowledge of the theorist; no one is truly a master of all the disciplines relevant to understanding and treating mental illness. I come from a systems neuroscience background—which means I study the functioning of general brain systems, such as the circuits responsible for the sense of touch—and I have no formal training in psychiatric medicine, pharmacology, or psychological brain science, and only a limited knowledge of molecular neuroscience. Nonetheless, the current theory (note: by 'current theory', I mean the set of theories contained in this book) is consistent with the general principles of these disciplines.

This book represents a synthesis of a large amount of information into a working theory of brain function that is relevant to treating mental illness. What are the origins of the theory? Some aspects come from my laboratory research, some from the scientific literature, some from the popular literature, some from my observations of many people over the years, and some from my experiences during the treatment of my own illness, bipolar disorder. I believe a reasonable theory with testable hypotheses is better than no theory at all for at least two reasons: 1) it affirms or eliminates one of the hypotheses, and 2) it stimulates discussion that may lead to improvement of the field of psychiatry. I want the reader to feel that he or she can make a contribution to this discussion also, by using common sense reasoning to analyze what I've written and thereby try to improve the theory.

The foundation of the current theory is that the brain chemicals serotonin (**ser**), norepinephrine (**nore**), and dopamine (**dop**)—the 'Big Three'—as well as the neural circuits they affect, provide the basis for not only understanding what causes most types of mental illness and how to treat those illnesses, but also for understanding basic human characteristics, personality traits, and our very perception of the world. A fundamental premise of the current theory is that the 'strengths'—by which I mean the chemical levels plus the sensitivity of the relevant brain circuits they affect—of these three chemical systems vary from individual to individual, mainly as a result of genetics, and that understanding approximately what the strengths are in a given individual is critical for treating mental illness and understanding mental health. Furthermore, it is assumed that the strengths or at least functioning of the three systems can be altered by environmental stimuli, such as stressors, and can be adjusted with psychiatric drugs and possibly talk therapy.

Part of the current theory is a rehashing of ideas that many researchers already had in the 1950s and 1960s, when many new types of psychiatric drugs were being synthesized and tested. In some respects it is a more general version of the chemical imbalance theories of depression and mania from the 1960s, which state that low brain levels of ser, nore, and dop cause depression, and that high levels cause mania, though many of the ideas are, to my knowledge, new. It is not meant to provide exhaustive information about any particular mental illness, but rather to examine some properties that prominent mental illnesses share.

Pop Philosophy

The current theory concerns both differences and similarities between people, particularly how different aspects of brain function affect our conscious experience of the world. In examining these issues, we are faced with popular philosophical problems, such as that language and all other forms of communication are limited in their ability to describe subjective conscious states, and this problem is additionally confounded by the possibility that a given individual may never experience a given state. For example, most people would say that we can't conceive of colors other than those we have experienced, and we can never know if others perceive those known colors in the same way that we do.

To return to the subject of mental illness, how will we know, for example, if one person is mildly depressed and another is not? And how will we know, for example, if the subjective experience produced by taking a psychiatric drug, such as Prozac, is similar among different people? Moreover, comparing this drug induced experience to our imagined effect of the drug prior to taking it, or trying to explain the effect to someone who has never tried it or even to someone who has, is certainly not straightforward and may not even be possible.

One objective source of information that we can use to address these problems is behavior. For understanding mental illness, this primarily includes both people's reports of their own experiences—including perceptual experiences—as well as our observations of those people. If behavior is similar among different people, we may infer not only what a given conscious experience is but also that the experience is similar among different people, though these inferences may not always be correct. Much of the current theory is, out of necessity, based on such inferences.

We can also address these philosophical problems by studying brain function. We can ask the question: to what extent can the brain be idealized to be the same, or at least very similar, among different people—or among all mammals, for example? If, for example, brain dysfunction is physiologically similar across individuals with the same (or similar) mental illness, then those different people may be experiencing similar conscious states. Most researchers would acknowledge that while each brain is unique in its exact structure and function, much of scientific research and medical practice, including psychiatry, assumes that there are common properties to the brain across individuals. For example, the diagnosis of a discrete number of mental illnesses (syndromes, such as schizophrenia) relies on some degree of commonality across individuals. I take the stance in this book that there are brain structural and functional commonalities that, while not being exactly the same across individuals, are similar enough that they produce similar conscious states that can be modulated, for example, by a given drug in similar ways.

Personality Differences

When there are significant, normal differences in the brain across individuals, I believe such differences evolved, by natural selection, to produce different personality traits, and that these differences are not frequently unique, but rather exist in clusters of other similar individuals. Given that there are significant and sometimes drastic differences in both personality and behavior between individuals, what accounts for the differences? The current theory's answer: variations in perception, originating from basic differences in brain function, form the basis of personality differences. If we could perceive the world the way others do, I think these differences would be obvious and profound. Indeed, philosophers and psychologists have long wondered whether we all perceive the world in a similar if not identical manner. The current theory indicates that people's perceptions—including their sensory perceptions—are, in fact, not identical.

The advent of widespread treatment of mental illness with drugs in the 1950s caused a revolution in psychiatry that continues today. As the eminent psychiatrist and author Peter Kramer has stated, one can 'listen to' the effect of a drug, assuming the validity of a particular brain mechanism of action for that drug (such as Prozac boosting ser), and from that action infer brain function both in the mentally ill brain and in the normal brain. Using this reasoning, part of the origin of the current theory lies with listening to the likely mechanisms of the drugs that are currently used to treat mental illness (pharmaceuticals), as well as drugs of abuse. Similarly, I have listened to personality across many people, because from it we can also infer brain function that, as I will describe in Chapter 12, may be directly related to Big Three function.

The *DSM-IV-TR*

The *Diagnostic and Statistical Manual of Mental Disorders* (current version: *DSM-IV-TR*), the standard diagnostic text of the American Psychiatric Association, probably represents the most widely read theoretical description of mental illness, though it is not very biological. I'm not trying to replace it with the current theory, but rather to supplement it. Nonetheless, that book is a caricature of the truth, even though it has probably identified the major forms of mental illness, and to an approximation, their clusters of symptoms.

In defense of the *Diagnostic and Statistical Manual*: it has represented important stages in our understanding of mental illness, namely that there are syndromes with constellations of symptoms, an idea which originated with eminent psychiatric researcher Emil Kraepelin. This idea is essentially correct, but the actual descriptions of particular illnesses in the current version are not completely correct; if they were then why do the authors keep changing the book? I believe there are almost certainly mental illnesses that have not been identified and accurately described, based solely on the incredible complexity of the brain. Moreover, some of the illnesses in the *Diagnostic and Statistical Manual* may have unidentified subtypes— such as atypical and typical bipolar disorder, which I describe in Chapter 10—and the lists of symptoms or characteristics will also probably change (possibly be expanded) somewhat as we come to understand these illnesses better. Nonetheless, abnormalities of the Big Three systems probably explain a significant number of the actual mental illnesses.

Origins of the Theory

The current theory originates from multiple sources of information: eminent psychiatric researcher C. Robert Cloninger's tri-dimensional (Big Three) personality model; ideas of my mentors, including Vernon Mountcastle and the late Kenneth Johnson, at the Johns Hopkins University Mind/Brain Institute on sensorimotor transformation and pattern recognition; Michael Norden's observation of ser strengthening drugs, such as Prozac, treating so many conditions and other ideas described in *Beyond Prozac*; Peter Kramer's observations of presumably weak ser/strong nore patients described in the epic *Listening to Prozac*, especially the observation that some patients can be made 'better than well' by Prozac; John Ratey's and Catherine Johnson's description of ubiquitous mild mental illness in *Shadow Syndromes*; Kay Jamison's observation of bipolar disorder being overrepresented among artists and other information about bipolar disorder in her books, *An Unquiet Mind, Touched with Fire*, and *Manic-Depressive Illness* (the latter book was co-authored by Frederick Goodwin); Samuel Barondes' various observations on the state of psychiatry in *Better than Prozac*; Raymond DePaulo's detailed information about depression and bipolar disorder in *Understanding Depression*, including the description of assortative mating; the Enneagram personality model, most informatively described by Don Riso; my own experiences with bipolar disorder, including the effects of drugs on me; my observations of normal and overtly mentally ill people throughout my life; and the scientific literature, including animal studies.

Regarding the scientific literature, there are often conflicting data on a single issue, partly because of the sheer number of studies that have been conducted, including studies of rodents and occasionally non-human primates. Indeed, the advanced studies of the brain in rodents and monkeys, primarily carried out in the last fifty years, are probably the most relevant to the current theory. I have avoided getting into he said, she said debates.

CHAPTER 1

A BRIEF HISTORY OF PSYCHIATRY

Major Points

• **Prior to the 1950s, drugs were not widely used to treat mental illnesses. Since then, many psychiatric drugs have been created, and many more are in the process of being created.**

• **In the 1960s, the Big Three neurotransmitters were shown to send connections from their brainstem neurons to widespread areas of the brain.**

• **Also in the 1960s, chemical imbalance theories of mania and depression were first put forth.**

Early History

Though psychiatric treatment has improved dramatically in the last fifty years with the advent of potent pharmaceutical drugs, the several thousand years of civilization leading up to that point relied upon crude and unproven methods to treat mental illness. The ancient Greeks and Romans developed the idea that four special bodily fluids, or humours, provide the basis of physical and mental health. These four humours were blood, black bile, yellow bile, and phlegm, where an excessive amount of black bile was associated with a melancholic temperament. To achieve balance of the four humours, and thereby gain optimal health, the ancients performed bloodletting when it was thought that an excessive amount of blood was contributing to an individual's poor health.

By the second millennium, knowledge of mental illness had not progressed substantially. The first mental asylum, Bethlem Royal Hospital (also known as Bedlam, which represents the origin of the commonly used expression for chaos), was opened in London in 1247, though it may not have represented progress for the mentally ill since those who were kept there were not treated nicely. Asylums were later built in many other countries, though treatment of their patients did not improve substantially until the 1800s when reformers such as Phillipe Pinel in France, William Tuke in England, and Dorothea Dix in the United States made great contributions to improving living conditions as well as attitudes toward the mentally ill.

By the 1940s, several new treatments were developed for mental illness: electroconvulsive therapy (ECT), insulin shock therapy, and frontal lobotomy, where the latter two are today considered barbaric and ineffective. ECT, which involves passing electrical current on the skull to induce a brief seizure in the brain, was barbaric in its early form because the patient was awake during the procedure, but today it is done safely under anesthesia and is very effective for treating severe depression and perhaps other forms of mental illness. Insulin shock therapy involved injecting a large dose of insulin into the patient to induce a seizure, and was used, probably unsuccessfully, to treat schizophrenia before the advent of antipsychotic medications. Frontal lobotomy, which involved surgically severing the prefrontal cortex from the rest of the brain, was said to sometimes have a calming effect on aggressive patients, but was otherwise ineffective in treating mental illness. Few lobotomies have been performed since the 1950s.

Kraepelin and Freud

By the beginning of the twentieth century, two European doctors and scholars, Emil Kraepelin and Sigmund Freud, would redefine the field of psychiatry altogether. Kraepelin, born in 1856, was a German psychiatrist who tried to make sense of the bewildering hundreds of mental disorders that had been named up to that point, by grouping illnesses together based on their characteristic patterns of symptoms. In this manner, he was the first to distinguish manic-depression (bipolar disorder) and schizophrenia as separate illnesses, each with distinct patterns of symptoms, though certain symptoms could be found in both illnesses. Kraepelin also thought that manic-depression tended to remain constant in severity throughout a patient's life, whereas schizophrenia tended to increase in severity throughout life.

Kraepelin's laboratory made important discoveries regarding the brain basis of Alzheimer's disease, and he thought that specific brain abnormalities caused the other mental illnesses, and that this would be proven in the future.

Sigmund Freud's fame far outstripped Kraepelin's, when both men were alive and to this day, though Kraepelin's ideas are probably the more accurate. Freud was also born in 1856, in his case in Austria, and was a neurologist by training. His greatest impact on the practice of psychiatry itself was creating psychoanalysis, which is a type of talk therapy in which the patient engages in free thought association and dream interpretation with the therapist to explore repressed or unconscious urges and conflicts, in order to improve the patient's psychological health. Psychoanalysis is rooted in several assumptions: 1) human development is strongly influenced by objects of sexual desire which change over time, particularly desire toward one's parents; 2) one's conscious mind often represses wishes that are then stored in the unconscious mind, and manifest themselves in dreams, Freudian slips, and psychological symptoms, such as neuroses (which is a catch-all term for mild mental illness); 3) neuroses are treatable through psychoanalysis by making the patient aware of his repressed, unconscious wishes.

Freud's ideas have not only had a profound effect on psychiatry, but also on our culture in general, by influencing books, films, politics, philosophy, and popular culture. However, there is little evidence that psychoanalysis is actually an effective treatment for any form of mental illness, and it has been widely criticized because of this. Indeed, just because an idea is interesting and impressive does not mean that it's true, or at least that it's completely true. There are still many psychiatrists who practice psychoanalysis, but this is becoming less common and the field may be in the process of dying.

Modern Medicine

Medicine in general, not just the field of psychiatry, has been improved tremendously since 1940, which is approximately when medical experiments, on both human subjects and animal models, began being performed in significant numbers. Thus, medicine became more strongly based in science. One of the landmark types of discoveries, for the purposes of this book, that occurred around this time was that neurons use particular chemicals, called neurotransmitters, to communicate with one another. One such neurotransmitter, serotonin (ser), was discovered in 1948, and by the 1960s the Big Three transmitters (ser), norepinephrine (nore), dopamine (dop) were each known to send connections from a relatively small number of neurons in the brainstem to widespread regions of the brain. Also, by the 1960s, many new psychiatric drugs, which in many cases affect the Big Three, were being created and marketed by the drug companies, and we'll discuss some of these drugs below.

Here Come the Drugs

In the early 1950s, scientists at a French drug company were trying to create a more effective sleeping pill when they happened upon a new compound that could not only calm manic patients, but also terminate psychosis (delusions and hallucinations) in patients with schizophrenia. They called the drug chlorpromazine, now better known as Thorazine, and it was the first effective antipsychotic medication. Other similar antipsychotic drugs were soon created.

Around this time, scientists at a Swiss drug company decided that they wanted to create an antipsychotic drug that could compete with chlorpromazine, so they synthesized similar molecules for testing in schizophrenic patients. They soon found one such new drug that did not treat schizophrenia, but, surprisingly, had a potent antidepressant effect in severely depressed patients. This drug became known as imipramine, and was the first in a class of drugs called the tricyclic antidepressants, so named for their three-ringed molecular structure. As you'll soon read, the tricyclic antidepressant desipramine has been a miracle drug for me.

Also in the 1950s, another Swiss drug company was testing a drug called iproniazid for the treatment of tuberculosis, when they noticed that the drug tended to have mood elevating properties. Iproniazid, later known as Parnate, became the first antidepressant in a class of drugs called the MAO inhibitors. The tricyclics became the more successful and broadly used antidepressants, since some of the MAO inhibitors can cause a lethal, high blood pressure crisis when the patient ingests certain cheeses and wines. However, milder versions of these drugs that do not have dietary restrictions are now used outside the United States.

By the late 1980s, another class of drugs, the ser reuptake inhibitors (SRIs), such as Prozac, had a dramatic effect on psychiatry. Since these drugs selectively boost ser, they were thought to be more specific in their effects than the tricyclics and MAO inhibitors, and devoid of most troublesome side effects. Due to their safety and the wide array of brain circuits affected by ser, the SRIs have been used to treat a variety of mental illnesses, including depression, anxiety, eating disorders, drug and alcohol abuse, and others. Indeed, the fact that the SRIs are effective in treating such a broad range of conditions has led to the hypothesis, put forth by Michael Norden and others, that most people have a ser deficiency.

In the 1990s and 2000s, several more antidepressants were produced that, like the tricyclics and MAO inhibitors, affect multiple

Big Three transmitter systems. These include the drugs Effexor, Cymbalta, and Remeron.

The treatment of bipolar disorder, similar to the treatment of unipolar depression, has seen great improvements since the 1950s with the advent of multiple mood stabilizing drugs. In 1949, the Australian psychiatrist John Cade discovered that the simple salt, lithium, has a calming effect on animals. He soon demonstrated that lithium can quell mania in patients with bipolar disorder, and by 1970 lithium was FDA approved in the United States for the treatment of bipolar disorder. Later, drugs that had been created to treat epilepsy, the anticonvulsants, also came in to broad use for the treatment of bipolar disorder. Among these are Tegretol and Depakote.

As mentioned earlier, older antipsychotics such as Thorazine, now known as typical antipsychotics, are effective in terminating bipolar mania and therefore have mood stabilizing properties. By the 1990s, a new wave of antipsychotics, known as the atypical antipsychotics, such as Zyprexa and Geodon, had hit the market. These drugs deactivate ser receptors strongly and dop receptors weakly, whereas the typical antipsychotics also deactivate ser receptors strongly but deactivate dop receptors strongly. Both classes of drugs can treat both schizophrenia and bipolar mania. Clozapine was the first atypical, and was actually available in Europe in the 1970s, though it is not that popular now because it can cause a rare blood disorder.

Chemical Imbalance Theories

As described above, by the 1960s there were Big Three boosting drugs, such as the tricyclics and the MAO inhibitors, that could effectively treat depression. This led the late Joseph Schildkraut at Harvard to propose, in 1965, the 'catecholamine hypothesis' of mood disorders, namely that a deficiency of nore (and possibly dop) causes depression. A corollary to this hypothesis is that excessive nore (and dop) causes mania. Similarly, in 1967, Alec Coppen proposed the 'indoleamine hypothesis' of mood disorders, namely that a deficiency of ser causes depression, with the corollary that excessive ser causes mania.

Combining the above two hypotheses, one arrives at what is known as the 'biogenic amine hypothesis' of mood disorders: deficiencies in ser, nore, and dop produce depression, whereas excessive amounts of the Big Three produce mania. However, no one, to my knowledge, has hypothesized that tweaking the Big Three to mid-range strengths treats nearly every type of mental illness, as in the current theory I am putting forth in this book.

A lesser known hypothesis of mood disorders, put forth by Janowsky and colleagues in 1972, is the 'cholinergic-adrenergic hypothesis' of mania and depression. It hypothesizes that strong acetylcholine/weak nore produces depression, whereas weak acetylcholine/strong nore produces mania. I discuss the neurotransmitter acetylcholine briefly in Chapter 17.

The *DSM*

The *Diagnostic and Statistical Manual of Mental Disorders* (*DSM*) is the standard mental illness diagnostic text of the American Psychiatric Association in the United States, and may be the most widely read psychiatric text in the world. Just as psychiatric drug treatment has changed greatly since the 1950s, so have the editions of the *DSM*. It has undergone five revisions (II, III, III-R, IV, IV-TR) since its first edition in 1952, and has ballooned from describing about 60 disorders to around 400 in the current version, IV-TR. The *DSM-V* is due to be published in 2011.

The *DSM* is based on the idea that particular mental illnesses have a characteristic set of symptoms, and that a particular illness in a particular person will exhibit a subset of those symptoms. One weakness of the book is that it is not very biological, and contains very little information about neuroscience or the brain.

Recent Advances

Brain imaging techniques, such as magnetic resonance imaging (MRI), positron emission tomography (PET), and single photon emission computed tomography (SPECT), have allowed psychiatric researchers to gain glimpses of the working brain in real time. MRI was developed in the 1970s and 1980s, and monitors changes in blood oxygenation that are thought to mirror changes in neural activity. PET monitors neural activity through the use of injected radioactive tracers that enter the brain, and SPECT is similar to PET in that it also relies on injected radioactive tracers interacting with the brain. All three techniques have potential to be applied to the everyday treatment of psychiatric patients, by monitoring the affected brain areas as well as how those areas are affected by drugs.

Other recent advances in psychiatric research include ongoing studies of the genetics of mental illness in both humans and animals, which have been facilitated by the recent complete mapping of the human genome. In addition, there are now ongoing studies of rodent models of depression, alcoholism, and schizophrenia.

The field of psychiatry has changed greatly in the last fifty years, especially due to the advent of widespread drug treatment and much greater knowledge of brain function. A wide range of scientific and medical techniques and disciplines are now impinging upon the field, and this makes major breakthroughs seem imminent. I believe the current theory described in this book represents one such breakthrough.

CHAPTER 2

MY CASE STUDY

Background

What follows is a summary of the events surrounding my successful drug treatment for bipolar disorder, including some of the amazing effects those drugs had on me. I'm including this case study for three primary reasons: 1) it illustrates a long journey similar to that which many people with mental illness must endure before eventually getting effective treatment; 2) some of my experiences provide the basis for parts of the current theory; and 3) it illustrates some useful principles for treating bipolar disorder and other mental illnesses, including a common sense problem solving approach that I believe should be applied by medical practitioners and their patients when treating mental illness.

The Case

One day in the summer of 1999, about four years into neuroscience graduate school at Johns Hopkins University in Baltimore, Maryland, I consulted a psychiatrist because I thought I might be suffering from clinical depression. The psychiatrist and I went over my list of symptoms, which included: depressed mood, persistent negative thinking, loss of appetite, and difficulty sleeping, with early morning awakenings. He concluded that I was indeed suffering from a bout of depression and decided to put me on Prozac. I faithfully took the proper dose every day, but after a month passed I still didn't feel any better, so my doctor decided to try Remeron, a newer antidepressant. I was on that drug for about six months, though it didn't do much to lift the depression, so I stopped taking it.

I went home to West Lafayette, Indiana for Christmas (1999)

vacation, and soon realized that I probably shouldn't return to the lab in Baltimore until I was feeling better. I found a local psychiatrist who put me on Effexor, which like Remeron was a fairly new antidepressant at the time. After a month on Effexor, I still had no response and decided to get a new doctor, partly because I was again starting to feel desperate to escape from the unrelentingly miserable depression. The new doctor decided to try Zoloft, which is a ser boosting drug like Prozac. After about two weeks on Zoloft, I began sleeping and feeling better, and soon I returned to Baltimore.

Though I had improved quite a bit (April 2000), I was still only sleeping six hours a night instead of my usual nine hours, and my personality seemed to have changed somewhat, as now I had a great interest in buying and selling things, couldn't sit still for very long, was filled with grand ideas and plans, was hyperactive and somewhat agitated, and couldn't seem to stop talking. I also noticed some clearly unpleasant side effects: my senses, especially my hearing, were less acute, and I seemed less emotionally sensitive. My new doctor in Baltimore concluded that I was exhibiting symptoms of hypomania, which is a mild form of mania, and therefore I had bipolar disorder, also known as manic-depressive illness. He suggested that I should be put on a mood stabilizing drug, such as lithium, but first decided to gradually reduce and then eliminate the Zoloft, and also added a small dose of the new mood stabilizing drug, Zyprexa, which deactivates dop and ser brain receptors. The hypomania soon subsided and then, after several weeks of feeling somewhat slowed down, I crashed into a depression that was just as severe as ever.

I then decided to check myself into the Johns Hopkins Hospital (October 2000). The doctors there confirmed the diagnosis of bipolar disorder and put me back on Zoloft to bring me out of the depression, and also added the mood stabilizing drug Depakote to prevent me from becoming hypomanic. After a few weeks on Depakote, I decided I didn't like the stuff because it felt like I had been hit over the head with a hammer, so I gradually stopped taking it. I also reduced the Zoloft to a very small dose, hoping this would prevent me from becoming hypomanic. It did not because soon I was exhibiting the same hypomanic symptoms as the first time on Zoloft.

Around this time I came up with the theory that I had a super high genetic level of ser, the brain chemical that Zoloft boosts, based both on my reaction to Zoloft and information I had gleaned from Peter Kramer's classic book, *Listening to Prozac*. I reasoned that Zoloft was making me hypomanic because it was making this chemical imbalance even more extreme, and that if I instead took an anti-depressant that boosts nore, a brain chemical of which I thought I had a super low genetic level, then the hypomania would not be triggered. Moreover, I reasoned that a nore boosting antidepressant, such as desipramine or nortriptyline, would not only *not* trigger hypomania, but also terminate Zoloft induced hypomania through reduction of the level of ser by nore (feedback inhibition). I ran this theory by my doctor who, though he didn't seem to believe it, was willing to let me test the theory by prescribing a small dose of nortriptyline to replace the Zoloft. Unfortunately, after several weeks on the nortriptyline it was apparent that the theory was incorrect, as I remained at least as hypomanic as on the Zoloft, though my senses seemed sharper. With this setback, I decided to follow the doctor's advice and try a low dose of the mood stabilizer lithium. Around this time, I also decided to leave graduate school with a Master's Degree and head back to Indiana.

I actually did feel a little better after the move (February 2001), though I was still somewhat hypomanic. Thinking that I might recover completely after some time in the new environment, I stopped taking the nortriptyline as well as the lithium. My new doctor prescribed a small dose of Zyprexa to quell the continuing mild hypomania, and this time on Zyprexa I noticed something new—like nortriptyline, it sharpened my senses, in contrast to the sensory deadening that Zoloft produced. However, by the middle of summer I crashed into another severe depression, much like I had after the first prolonged hypomanic episode on Zoloft in the summer of 2000. I checked myself into a hospital in Lafayette and asked the doctor to put me on a super high dose of Zyprexa, which I reasoned wouldn't make me hypomanic and may boost my low level of nore by inhibiting my high level of ser. The doctor agreed to try the massive dose, also adding Wellbutrin, which is an unusual antidepressant in that it usually does not induce hypomania.

Soon I was released from the hospital (summer 2001) even though I was still in pretty bad shape. I limped along for a few months on this pair of drugs, but the depression only lifted slightly. My doctor wanted to put me back on Zoloft, but I vetoed this in favor of the nore boosting antidepressant desipramine. I still didn't believe that I was truly bipolar, instead maintaining the theory that I had a super high level of ser and a low level of nore, and that boosting nore alone would cause the depression to lift and not make me hypomanic. Five weeks after starting on a low dose of desipramine, I weaned myself of the Wellbutrin and the massive dose of Zyprexa, viewing these drugs as no longer necessary; the depression had now lifted and I thought I was cured. Unfortunately, after a few more weeks on desipramine I realized that the depression had given way to an unpleasant hypomania. Now, for the first time realizing that maybe I really was bipolar, I consulted the doctor and he put me back on a moderate dose of Zyprexa and kept me on the low dose of desipramine, and within a few days I was much less hypomanic.

I spent the next year (early 2002 to early 2003) tweaking the doses of both desipramine and Zyprexa. Too much desipramine made me feel like a zombie (which I call the 'zombie effect') and also induced rapid, unpleasant mood cycling; too much Zyprexa caused a multi-year depression-like effect that I call the 'brain freeze', from which I'm still recovering. It took only a slightly higher dose of Zyprexa than I'm currently on to produce the brain freeze, and it's possible that other drugs besides Zyprexa can cause a similar brain freeze. I was only on the higher dose of Zyprexa for three weeks, during which time I had a headache and felt tired most of the time, which I now realize were signs of the developing brain freeze, but at the time I thought these were just normal side effects of the higher dose of the drug that would soon go away. The main symptoms of the brain freeze that I first noticed were that my ability to think, remember things, and express myself were greatly impaired.

In summer 2003, I went back to graduate school at Johns Hopkins to finish my Ph.D., a testament to the partial success of my treatment. During this first year of the brain freeze, I didn't recognize that my low energy, poor appetite, headache, and general malaise had been caused by the high dose of Zyprexa—I instead thought I was suffering from a prolonged illness of some kind. Accordingly, I visited a general practitioner (April 2004) and obtained a prescription for a potent antibiotic, Zithromax, which I took over the course of five days. Unfortunately, the Zithromax appeared to interfere with the breakdown of desipramine, because I soon became both markedly hypomanic and 'zombiefied'. The hypomania lasted about a week and then I crashed back into a significant depression, which lasted about a month. After that, something amazing happened: I got slightly hypomanic again, but this time the characteristics of the hypomania were different and glorious. My perception of the world was altered such that everything seemed like a colored cartoon (as in Andy Behrman's book, *Electroboy*) in which just about everything seemed thrillingly interesting and women, especially their faces, seemed much more attractive, with pretty ones looking like goddesses (I mean their actual physical appearance was different)—effects that can't be described as merely sensory sharpening, but rather as perceptual changes. This strange and wonderful bout of hypomania, which made the whole year worth living, only lasted a few days, and then the usual, milder depressions and hypomanias returned, though I also noticed that the hypomanias now tended to be accompanied by arrhythmia (irregular heartbeat).

As summer (2004) continued, I gradually started feeling worse and then identified the cause: I had been using old desipramine that was apparently losing its potency, so I switched back to new desipramine in September. Then, once again, something amazing happened: whereas before the world seemed stale, flat, and unprofitable, it now seemed full of life and color. Once again, women looked extraordinarily beautiful, and everything else seemed inviting and extremely interesting—even though I wasn't necessarily very hypomanic. In other words, it was as if this is the way the world seems *all the time* to someone who isn't depressed (or, as I'll describe in Chapter 11, 'expanded dysthymic'), particularly since the brain freeze was subsiding.

This wonderful effect lasted until early October, at which point I crashed into another mild depression and started sleeping a lot—at first I thought that I was sick again. But after the depression lasted a few more months, I realized that this might be a wintertime, seasonal depression, superimposed upon mood cycling. So I decided to try bright light therapy—the standard treatment for seasonal affective disorder (SAD)—with a fluorescent light box. I also remained on my previous doses of Zyprexa and desipramine. The light box produced a few unpleasant side effects: cold and shaky hands, and an upset gut—consistent with it boosting ser in the brain and throughout the rest of the body, though I didn't think so at the time—but after a few weeks of sitting in front of it for thirty minutes every morning, I began feeling better. I continued using the light box throughout the winter, and by the beginning of April (2005), my brain seemed to begin undergoing a transitional state out of the wintertime depression. By the start of May, the arrhythmia returned, which had been absent throughout the winter, accompanied by marked and unpleasant hypomania—it actually seemed more like a mixed state (which is a mixture of hypomania and depression), with mood cycling every few days. At this point I realized that the light box was probably just boosting ser, since the hypomania wasn't that much different than the Zoloft induced hypomanias of several years before, so I quit the light box cold turkey, gradually recovering over the next few months from a state of mild depression, and that gets us up to the present day (July 2005).

Typically now I'm slightly hypomanic for a day or two, slightly depressed for the next day or two, and the cycle then repeats. I've reached the conclusion that I'm on the optimal doses of both Zyprexa and desipramine, both of which have essentially no side effects, other than mild arrhythmia presumably caused by desipramine, though I expect mild mood cycling will always be present. Both during hypomanias and depressions, this combination of drugs now clearly produces sensory sharpening, increases my level of interest in most things, heightens my emotions, and affects perceptual phenomena such as women seeming more beautiful or music sounding altered in a more interesting manner—effects that I definitely perceive as positive. Just how dramatic these changes will become, particularly after the brain freeze subsides completely, remains to be seen. Even if things don't get any better, in some ways I seem to have come to life for the first time, and the Big Three drugs if used properly may essentially do the same for many other people.

Conclusions that can be drawn from this case study (in chronological order):

1) A person may seem to have unipolar depression rather than bipolar disorder until an antidepressant induces mania or hypomania, 'unmasking' the bipolar disorder. In retrospect, the person may realize that he had mild hypomanias, as well as depressions, before taking antidepressants, especially in the case of bipolar II disorder.

2) A person may have no response or a partial response to several antidepressants, while having a robust response to others. Moreover, a person can respond to one drug within a class (say, SRIs—the ser reuptake inhibitors, such as Prozac and Zoloft, that boost the level of ser) and not to another drug in the same class.

3) Just because a particular antidepressant makes a bipolar depressed person hypomanic, doesn't mean it's the right one for him (or that he should be on an antidepressant at all). Moreover, a drug that is excellent for one person may be terrible or useless for someone else.

4) A newer drug is not necessarily better than an older drug, both in its average effect on many people and also for a given individual.

5) Changing the strengths of ser or nore with drugs can alter personality traits.

6) In some individuals, drugs that strengthen ser may deaden the senses and emotions, whereas drugs that strengthen nore may heighten the senses and emotions. Moreover, drugs that weaken ser (such as Zyprexa) may also heighten the senses and emotions. These effects may occur most prominently when the individual has genetically strong ser and weak nore—as in my case—with the drugs serving to counteract this chemical imbalance.

7) Periods of hypomania or mania are typically followed by a crash into depression, with the magnitude of the depression proportional to the magnitude of the preceding hypomania or mania. So perhaps the best strategy when treating bipolar disorder with an

antidepressant and a mood stabilizer is to maximize the dose of the mood stabilizer and minimize the dose of the antidepressant, in an effort to avoid pronounced hypomanias that are followed by pronounced depressions.

8) Very low doses of a drug can still be effective for a given person, and too high a dose of a drug can be a bad thing, since there seems to be a limit to the extent to which the brain can adjust to changes in Big Three strengths. Moreover, the effect of being on two drugs—in my case, Zyprexa and desipramine—at the same time can be different both in character and in magnitude than the effect of either drug alone. In other words, the net effect is different than the sum of the parts—what an engineer might call a 'nonlinearity'.

9) Adjusting the strengths of ser and nore with drugs in bipolar persons may affect the characteristics of hypomanias and depressions. Moreover, bringing the strengths of ser and nore closer to optimal, mid-range values (i.e., The Adjustment) may make the hypomanias more pleasant and depressions less unpleasant.

10) Without taking drugs or even while taking the existing drugs, bipolar (especially bipolar II) persons may always experience mood cycling. The best treatment strategy may be to use the existing drugs to minimize the magnitude—though not necessarily the frequency—of the hypomanias and depressions.

11) Mania/hypomania and perhaps depression, whether influenced by drugs or not, may produce perceptual changes, such as altering perception of the physical appearance of other people.

12) Heart pain or arrhythmia may be indicative of systemic nore changes; gut malfunctioning—and possibly cold hands, given the effect of ser on smooth muscle tissue such as that which lines blood vessels—may be indicative of systemic ser changes.

13) A change of scenery, activities, friends, even significant other, probably won't stop overt mental illness—these things may help coping, however.

14) Zyprexa may be anti-Zoloft in that these drugs may have opposing effects; more generally, atypical antipsychotics such as Zyprexa may be anti-SRI.

15) The 'brain freeze' may have been specific to ser, nore, or dop, or some combination of the three, including adjusting ser and nore in opposite strength directions with drugs.

16) If bright light therapy boosted nore and the nore strength had not dropped during the wintertime, it should have produced a zombie effect in me, but it did not. Moreover, I had no arrhythmia during the wintertime. Both of these observations are consistent with my wintertime depression being caused by a decrease in nore strength.

17) It was as if the brain freeze, or more generally depression itself, affects a number of perceptual traits simultaneously, such as sensory perception, rate and subject matter of thought, emotion, mood, drive states such as hunger and thirst, memory, and sexual potency—integrated in the brain in some as yet undiscovered manner (in other words, a 'neural integrator'). The basis for the neural integrator could be common input from the Big Three transmitters to multiple brain areas, or a single brain area

interconnected with many other areas. More generally, the neural integrator may exist in every brain, whether the person suffers from overt mental illness or not.

18) It's possible for a given individual to become much better than well by adjusting ser and nore closer to mid-range, optimal strengths (i.e., The Adjustment).

CHAPTER 3

GENERAL CHARACTERISTICS OF BRAIN FUNCTION

Major Points

- **Research conducted on the sensory systems of the macaque monkey gives clues about the causes of mental illness in the human brain.**

- **Illustrates the concepts of serial and parallel processing, sensorimotor transformation, pattern recognition, localization of function, encoding of information, attentional processes, cortical plasticity, and equilibria/steady-state processes, all of which are relevant to mental health.**

A biological theory of mental illness must, I believe, be in some ways a general theory of brain function, partly because a wide range of brain circuits are involved in mental illness. However, it is far beyond the scope of this book—and beyond the scope of human knowledge—to create a working model of the brain that describes its complete functioning in detail. Nonetheless, scientists have already gleaned data that provide clues to some of the brain's basic functional properties. I'd now like to touch upon some of these properties that may be important for understanding the **Big Three** brain chemicals (**ser**, **nore**, and **dop**) and their circuits in particular, and mental illness in general.

The current theory is based on the hypothesis that the electrical properties of the brain produce the mind, and that the brain is responsible for our conscious mental states. Ideally we will someday understand brain function on multiple levels, from molecule, to neuron, to interaction of millions of neurons in complex brain circuits, to behavior.

Sensory Systems

First let's touch upon the organization of sensory systems of the brain, since monkey neurophysiologists, who study the functional properties of neurons, know more about these areas of the brain than other areas more directly related to most mental illnesses. By understanding how the brain's sensory systems are organized, we may glean information regarding how the rest of the brain is organized, including the rest of the Big Three circuits.

There are multiple, interconnected cortical (where 'cortical' refers to the cerebral hemispheres of the brain) areas for processing information from each of the five senses; this is most well established for vision, hearing, and touch. The macaque monkey visual system has 30+ separate, interconnected cortical areas, and other macaque sensory systems have multiple areas, too. For each sense, the multiple areas are wired together in a hierarchical manner, with early areas feeding into later areas in a streamlike manner. These early areas have lower level functions that more faithfully represent sensory stimuli and respond to simple physical features of stimuli—in other words, they contain close to a point-for-point, or isomorphic, representation of the sensory input—whereas higher order sensory areas less faithfully respond to simple features and more so to particular combinations of features, giving rise to the ability to recognize objects. Exactly how this information transformation occurs is not well understood. For example, lower order visual areas contain neurons that respond to bars of light, whereas higher order areas contain neurons that respond to complex objects such as faces, though it is unclear how such neurons affect our perception of faces. (Recall that my perception of women's faces was altered during certain periods of hypomania, and now they seem more beautiful than before all the time!)

Within each sensory system, the brain may carry out integration of multiple sources of information. For example, in vision, there is a ventral stream of cortical areas, located near the bottom of the brain, devoted to processing what an object looks like, and a dorsal stream, located near the top of the brain, devoted to processing where the object is. Somehow these two types of information, 'what' and 'where', must be reunited to form our overall percept of a given object, and this is known as the binding problem—it is a central problem in sensory neurophysiology. The binding problem can also be framed in a more general manner: for example, are mood, emotion, thought, sensation, drive states such as hunger and thirst, and movement combined somehow to form our unified perception of reality, or instead are these entities processed in parallel and not reunited? Either way, the Big Three appear to affect such neural integration in a fundamental manner (see My Case Study). Indeed, mental illnesses such as major depression, bipolar disorder, schizophrenia, and anxiety disorders affect many of these traits simultaneously.

Brain sensory systems also contain examples of both serial and parallel processing, much like a circuit board in a household appliance. For example, the cortical streams devoted to the different senses are to some degree parallel to one another, and there are even parallel subpathways within the sensory cortical pathways, such as the visual ventral and dorsal streams, whereas each stream itself represents primarily serial processing. On a smaller physical scale, there are separate neuronal layers and different neuronal types within a given cortical area, with complex patterns of connectivity, including convergence and divergence, within and across layers, and such connectivity can be thought of as both serial and parallel. Primary visual cortex (area V1) is an example of parallel circuits (representing the form, color, and motion of objects) within one cortical area, as are multiple groups of neurons within such brain areas as the thalamus, amygdala, and hypothalamus. So there can be multiple circuits coursing through a particular brain area, and a single neuron can itself be part of multiple circuits. So if a given mental illness affects multiple brain areas, it may be affected by multiple serial or parallel processes.

What is the brain doing with all of this sensory information that it is processing? One of the principal purposes may be to perform sensorimotor transformations, a subject elaborated upon by my mentors at the Johns Hopkins Mind/Brain Institute such as Vernon Mountcastle and the late Kenneth Johnson. Such transformations can be thought of as stimulus-response functions. Even very simple organisms, such as bacteria and plants, engage in sensorimotor transformations. For example, some bacteria 'sense' a certain nutrient in their environment, and then swim ('motor') toward the region of highest concentration of that nutrient. In vertebrates, the spinal cord takes part in elementary sensorimotor transformations. For example, when certain muscles in the leg are stretched—as in when a doctor gently taps a patient below the knee with a mallet to test her reflexes—sensory neurons send an electrical impulse through the nerve to the spinal cord, and then motor neurons in the spinal cord send an electrical impulse back to the muscle that causes the leg to move such that it counteracts the stretch. In the human brain, sensori-motor transformations are much more complex, where very roughly speaking, the back of the brain is sensory and the front of the brain is motor. For example, in addition to sensory input, the brain must integrate mood, emotion, thought, drive states such as hunger and thirst, and memory to produce movement. We are not conscious of many aspects of this integration. We can also think about these processes in terms of motivation, goal directedness, and reinforcement of behavior—all of which are affected by mental illness. The brain may operate via a working, hierarchical plan that is updated continuously, in which conscious and unconscious states are integrated to produce goal-directed behavior.

In order for the brain to perform sensorimotor transformations, it must be able to recognize particular sensory stimuli. Indeed, the brain has a powerful capacity for such pattern recognition, at which it is usually successful in spite of variability in the location, size, and lighting of a given object, for example. Pattern recognition may indeed be the principal function of the multiple sensory cortical areas that comprise each sensory stream, or more generally the principal function of many of the Big Three circuits. The most well studied example of pattern recognition is visual object recognition, which sensory neurophysiologists are currently investigating in the ventral stream of cortical areas. The circuits that mediate transient anxiety, face recognition, sense of aesthetics, appreciation of music, and sexual attraction may all be performing types of pattern recognition. In contrast, some circuits may not require particular patterns of input for activation, such as those that mediate mood. Mental illnesses can in some ways be seen as disturbances in various pattern recognition circuits. In addition, researcher C. Robert Cloninger's Big Three functions, which we will discuss in Chapter 12, appear to be examples of pattern recognition.

Another note on brain sensory systems: they may not be exclusively sensory in function. Cortical neurophysiological studies in animals have shown that the brain actually exhibits incomplete localization of function: 'sensory' areas are partly motor, partly memory, for example. Likewise, 'motor' areas are partly sensory. Even prefrontal cortex, which is probably primarily involved in thinking, responds to sensory input. So there is predominant localization of function, but it may not be absolute in that different areas of the brain appear to have overlapping functions. This implies that there may not be brain areas devoted exclusively to processing mood or other Big Three functional properties.

Information Processing

How do the brain sensory systems, or other brain areas, actually represent the information that they are processing? Well, the brain may actually employ multiple means for encoding information. Probably the most widely accepted code among neurophysiologists and theorists is that brain circuits are activated by the *average* action potential (electrical impulse) firing rates of their neurons. Another possibility is that the precise timing of firing of action potentials encodes the information. In either case, it is the electrical properties of neurons that are responsible for our perception of reality, as well as for the manifestation of mental illness.

Action potentials are an example of an all-or-none (thresholded) phenomenon, in that a neuron either produces a given one or it does not—there is no middle ground. In other words, a thresholded phenomenon has a simple, abrupt yes or no answer—there is no maybe. For example, in a U.S. presidential election, a candidate either wins or does not win the office; she's never 'sort of the president'. The brain actually contains examples of both thresholded phenomena and continua, where the latter are things that exist as a smooth range, such as the temperature of the air. The effects of the Big Three on a given cortical circuit may be continuous, thresholded, or both. Moreover, mental illnesses themselves may be characterized by both continuous and thresholded processes.

Regardless of how the brain encodes information, it has a limited capacity to process that information, and what you happen to be paying attention to can affect what is processed. Attention can be subdivided into top down versus bottom up processes. Top down processes are those in which we are consciously selecting something to pay attention to, such as a television show we are watching, whereas bottom up processes seize attention, as in a sudden, loud noise, and thereby gain access to awareness. Certain mental illnesses, such as attention deficit hyperactivity disorder (ADHD) and bipolar disorder, are characterized by marked impairment of attentional processes.

While the brain has a profound, though limited capacity to process information, it also can adapt to that information by exhibiting plasticity, which is the ability to change itself, at both the single neuron and general brain systems (organization of millions of neurons) levels, such as in the formation of long-term memories. In the last decade it was discovered that the adult brain is even capable of producing new neurons. Moreover, the adult brain can be modified by various environmental inputs such as Big Three drugs—and including sensory stimuli, of course—possibly in complex ways that can produce sustained effects. Furthermore, the developing brain exhibits critical periods, which are windows of opportunity that close after a certain amount of time, for the acquisition of normal adult properties, such as language and vision.

Finally, the brain contains examples of equilibria/steady-state processes, which are processes that are constant over time. For example, the level of water in a particular lake is in a state of equilibrium if the total amount of water going into it and the total amount going out of it are equal, thereby leaving the level unchanged over time. Mental illnesses may represent disturbances in brain equilibrium. The brain also contains examples of short-term (acute) and long-term (chronic) processes, including at the level of the single neuron. Short-term processes take place immediately, and long-term processes take place over a longer period of time and may even last indefinitely. Big Three drugs produce both short-term and long-term effects, though these effects may sometimes only be perceived as long-term, such as an antidepressant taking effect after two weeks.

CHAPTER 4

ENTER THE BIG THREE

Major Points

• **The Big Three neurotransmitter systems (ser, nore, and dop)—and drugs that affect them—turn many brain processes on and off.**

• **Ser and nore form a neurochemical yin and yang, and are the principal players in mental illness, with dop having a less important role.**

• **There is a single level of each of the Big Three throughout the brain, and the molecular receptors for ser and nore are ordinarily saturated.**

• **Introduces the concept of a 'strength' for each of the Big Three, which means the level of the transmitter plus the sensitivity of the circuitry to that level.**

• **Contrasts mental illness caused by abnormal Big Three strengths and that caused by dysfunctional Big Three systems.**

The current theory is based on the functions of three brain chemicals—serotonin (ser), norepinephrine (nore), and dopamine (dop), which I have referred to as the Big Three—and the circuits they affect. These are not the only chemicals in the brain, but perhaps they are the most relevant to treating mental illness and understanding mental health. Indeed, most psychiatric drugs with known mechanisms of action achieve their effects by altering one or more of these three chemical systems.

The goal of this book is not to describe how the brain works in detail, but rather how the Big Three turn some of its functions on and off. By analogy, while we may not know in detail how a computer works, we definitely know some of the things it can do, including that we can influence some of its inputs and outputs—by typing on the keyboard, clicking the mouse, and turning the power on and off. Doing so affects the internal circuitry of the computer in some manner—and we may speculate as to how—and we can observe some of the corresponding outputs, such as on the video monitor. Likewise, we can adjust the strengths of the Big Three with drugs, and observe the effects on ourselves and on others.

Fundamentals of a Synapse

The Big Three are actually neurotransmitters, or substances that neurons use to communicate with one another across gaps called synapses (see Figure 1). Before we continue, let's discuss some of the fundamental properties of synapses, where many of these properties are shown in Figure 1. A typical synapse consists of the gap between a so-called presynaptic neuron and a so-called postsynaptic neuron. The presynaptic neuron is sending a message to the postsynaptic neuron, which is receiving the message. The message is carried by the neurotransmitter, which is a simple brain chemical that is stored in little packets called vesicles inside the presynaptic neuron. When an electrical impulse called an action potential reaches the end of the presynaptic neuron, neurotransmitter is released into the synapse and it floats around, binding to receptors on the outside of the postsynaptic neuron (and even to receptors on the outside of the presynaptic neuron, which are called autoreceptors and can affect the rate at which the transmitter is released) in a key and lock manner. When the neurotransmitter binds to the postsynaptic receptors, this typically

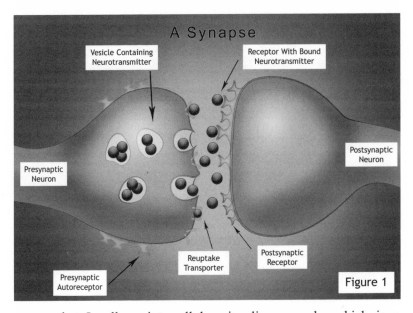

A Synapse

Vesicle Containing Neurotransmitter

Receptor With Bound Neurotransmitter

Postsynaptic Neuron

Presynaptic Neuron

Presynaptic Autoreceptor

Reuptake Transporter

Postsynaptic Receptor

Figure 1

starts what I call an intracellular signaling cascade, which is a series of chemical reactions that take place inside the postsynaptic neuron that may help trigger an action potential with which it can communicate with the next neuron. Meanwhile, the neurotransmitter is pumped back inside the presynaptic neuron by molecules called reuptake transporters, thereby terminating the signal. In addition, a molecule called monoamine oxidase (MAO) can break down the transmitter and thereby deactivate it. For each of the Big Three, there are multiple types ('subtypes') of postsynaptic receptors, where each subtype may affect the postsynaptic neuron in a different manner, and may be present in different types of neurons and in different circuits in the brain.

Now let's examine some of the effects that Big Three drugs can have on a synapse. In general, these drugs can either affect the level of the neurotransmitter in the synapse through a variety of means; or instead activate or deactivate the postsynaptic receptors directly, thereby mimicking the effects of the transmitter. Some drugs instead enter the postsynaptic neuron and affect intracellular signaling cascades directly, and I call these intracellular drugs.

Big Three drugs that affect the level of the transmitter in the synapse do so by: increasing or decreasing presynaptic transmitter release by activating (i.e., agonizing) or deactivating (i.e., antagonizing or blocking) presynaptic autoreceptors; increasing or decreasing transmitter reuptake by binding to the reuptake transporter; or decreasing breakdown of the transmitter by binding to monoamine oxidase (MAO). For example, the drug clonidine activates nore presynaptic autoreceptors and thereby decreases the release of nore into the synapse. Prozac deactivates the ser reuptake transporter—hence the name ser reuptake inhibitor (SRI)—and thereby allows more ser to build up in the synapse. The drug Parnate, which was mentioned earlier, decreases the activity of the MAO molecule—hence the name MAO inhibitor—and thereby allows the Big Three to build up in the synapse. Big Three drugs that increase the level of the transmitter in the synapse should strengthen that transmitter system, and drugs that decrease the level should weaken that transmitter system.

Big Three drugs can also mimic the effects of the neurotransmitters themselves by binding directly to postsynaptic receptors, and either activating them (which is what transmitters do), or deactivating them. For example, the drug Zyprexa deactivates several postsynaptic receptors, including the dop D2 receptor and the ser 5HT_2A receptor, thereby weakening both dop and ser neurotransmission. Big Three drugs that activate postsynaptic receptors should strengthen that transmitter system, and drugs that deactivate postsynaptic receptors should weaken that transmitter system.

Modulatory Neurotransmitters

Most neuroscientists think of the Big Three, especially ser and nore, as *modulatory* neurotransmitters, since they are dispersed throughout many regions of the brain and may have very general effects on brain function, where the simplest form of neural modulation may be activation or inactivation of circuits, like an 'on and off' light switch or the volume dial on a radio. For each of the Big Three, a relatively small number of neurons located in groups (nuclei) in the brainstem are connected with widespread regions of the brain, and these neurons release the neurotransmitter to modulate the responses of millions of other neurons. (In contrast, other neurotransmitters, such as glutamate and GABA, are released in a very precise, localized manner, usually helping neighboring neurons communicate.) Because of their connections with many regions of the brain, the Big Three are poised to affect a number of brain functions, including mood, emotion, thought, sensation, learning and memory, movement, sleep, drive states, sexuality (sexual drive/orientation), and disease.

The current theory hypothesizes that ser and nore (the Big Two, if you will) are the principal players in mental illness, and that dop has a less important role. As we shall see, ser and nore can be thought of as a neurochemical yin and yang, since many of their effects on the brain are directly opposed. More is known about ser than about nore, partly because of the widespread use of ser strengthening drugs—the serotonin reuptake inhibitors (SRIs), such as Prozac and Zoloft. In this book I repeatedly refer to the 'strengths' of the Big Three, by which I mean the extracellular, or outside the brain cell, level of the neurotransmitter in the brain plus the sensitivity of the circuits it affects to that level. (The functioning of the Big Three presynaptic brainstem neurons in releasing these neurotransmitters therefore also plays a critical role in strength.) Based on my research I believe that different people have different genetic strengths of the Big Three, and that these strengths can be affected by drugs and other environmental factors, such as stress. A central point in this book is that the immediate future of psychiatry should involve using drugs to adjust the brain strengths of ser and nore—and in some cases, dop—closer to optimal, mid-range degrees (i.e., The Adjustment). This could improve quality of life, possibly dramatically, both for people with overt mental illness and even for people who are considered normal. In other words, when one of the Big Three is too strong or too weak, the brain is in many ways not functioning in the best possible manner, and this situation worsens when more than one of the Big Three is too strong or too weak.

Single, Systemic Levels

The current theory puts forth the idea that there is a single, systemic level of each of the Big Three, throughout the brain, and for ser and nore, that correlates with the level throughout the rest of the body. For example, in a given person I don't think there are very different levels of ser in different areas of the brain. And since ser is also found in the gut, I think someone with a high level of ser in the brain will also have a high level of ser in the gut. Likewise, someone with a high level of nore in the brain will also have a high level of nore in the heart.

In support of this single, systemic level hypothesis, I think certain personality traits (see Chapter 7), which may be affected by different Big Three circuits, tend to coexist within a given person. This coexistence is consistent with a particular level of ser, for example, having a consistent effect on these different brain circuits. The single, systemic hypothesis is also consistent with My Case Study, which indicates that the brain level of nore (in making me hypomanic) correlates with the heart level of nore (in simultaneously causing my arrhythmia), and that the brain level of ser (in having an antidepressant effect during my bright light therapy) correlates with the gut level of ser (in simultaneously upsetting my gut). This hypothesis is also consistent with the neural integrator idea discussed in Chapter 2. However, it does not imply that everyone's circuitry is equally sensitive to the given level, or that the sensitivity of different circuits within a brain must correlate with one another, though I think this latter point tends to be the case as well. For these reasons, knowing the blood or even cerebrospinal fluid (CSF) levels of the Big Three, which researchers have been measuring for years, may not reliably indicate Big Three strengths, since one could have a low level of ser, for example, but with extremely sensitive circuitry to that level, resulting in a strong ser system that couldn't have been predicted from the level alone.

An alternative hypothesis is that there are different levels of the Big Three in different brain areas or circuits, affecting a number of traits in an independent manner. For example, there may be a high level of ser in the prefrontal cortex, affecting thought patterns in a particular way, whereas there may be a low level of ser in sensory cortex, affecting sensory perception in a different way. If this alternative hypothesis turns out to be true—and it is widely believed among researchers and psychiatrists, though I am confident that it is not true—it will take a lot longer for us to figure out how the Big Three work. Along these lines, I'm not sure psychiatric researchers want to hypothesize that there are single, systemic Big Three levels because it may be bad for getting grants!

Saturation of Ser and Nore, with a Safety Factor

The ser and nore (and possibly dop) levels seem to build as the day wears on, and are reabsorbed during sleep. This may explain the diurnal (within the day) fluctuation in mood during some cases of major depression, as well as the antidepressant effect of sleep deprivation. This is also consistent with experimental evidence indicating that brainstem ser and nore neurons actively fire action potentials (and thereby release neurotransmitter) while animals are awake, fire less frequently during NREM (non-rapid eye movement) sleep, and don't fire at all during REM sleep.

It also appears that the ser and nore postsynaptic circuitry is ordinarily saturated, or filled to capacity, with these two neuro-transmitters, whereas the dop circuitry is not. This means that somewhere in the circuitry raising the level of ser or nore doesn't have any immediate effect, whereas raising the level of dop does have an immediate effect. For example, ser or nore boosting antidepressants generally don't have a noticeable effect for two weeks, whereas dop boosting drugs, such as cocaine and amphetamine, have immediate effects.

The concept of what an engineer might call a 'safety factor' applies here: the level of ser and nore *exceeds* the point of saturation of the receptor population in the postsynaptic circuitry by a certain amount. This means that all of the receptors are bound with transmitter, in a key and lock manner, but there's also some additional transmitter floating around. In other words, if the brain was 'engineered' to operate with saturated postsynaptic receptors, it's not surprising that it also has some extra transmitter floating around as a 'safety' measure, to ensure that the receptors are indeed saturated. The point of saturation plus a safety factor may occur in the receptor population at the first postsynaptic synapse, inside the first postsynaptic neuron (involving signaling cascades inside the neuron), or further along in the circuitry. Ser or nore level boosting antidepressants may upregulate the postsynaptic circuitry by increasing the number or sensitivity of postsynaptic receptors or intracellular signaling cascades after two weeks, while maintaining a safety factor. In other words, the ser or nore circuitry has been strengthened, and the brain may maintain the safety factor throughout and after this process.

To return to the example of diurnal (within a day) mood fluctuation in some cases of major depression: perhaps stressors (which may deplete the levels of the Big Three) have eliminated the safety factor, while the postsynaptic receptor population has remained the same or diminished somewhat, and therefore mood increases as the day wears on because the unsaturated receptor population is receiving gradually increasing ser or nore input (since, as mentioned earlier in the chapter, ser and nore build as the day wears on). Different ser and nore safety factor levels may make certain people susceptible to mental illness. In other words, the smaller the safety factor the more likely that stressors will trigger mental illness.

Dysfunction and Stress

Some cases of mental illness may not be caused by abnormal strengths of the Big Three at all, but instead by a dysfunctional Big Three system. In other words, the normal functioning of the Big Three circuitry has been disrupted and needs to be reset to a healthy state. It could be that the dysfunction is due to a change in Big Three level without the postsynaptic circuitry adjusting to the change; in other words, a difference between actual level and expected level. For example, depression may in some cases involve a depleted level of one of the Big Three that the brain was not 'expecting', resulting in dysfunction in its circuitry. Electroconvulsive therapy (ECT) may reset dysfunctional circuits without altering Big Three levels, since it can be effective both at treating depression and mania, two conditions that may be caused by low or high Big Three levels, respectively. Another way to reset the circuitry may be to adjust Big Three strengths with level altering drugs, such as certain antidepressants.

A few more words about stress and mental illness. Stress may be a precipitating factor in many—but probably not all—cases of overt mental illness. The brainstem ser and nore neurons release these two neurotransmitters in response to certain types of stress, though exactly which types of stimuli cause these neurons to respond is an area of active research. If certain types of stressors cause massive release of ser or nore, then soon afterward there may be depleted release and diminished synaptic levels of these neurotransmitters, a phenomenon that a neuro-scientist would call postexcitatory depression. The brain may 'think' that it still has the old level of the transmitter, and therefore there is dysfunction: a difference between the expected level and the actual level. In addition, there can be long-term activation of the body's stress coping machinery—including activation of the hypothalamic-pituitary-adrenal (HPA) group of brain areas and release of the stress hormone cortisol—

during major depression and perhaps other types of mental illness.

Continua Versus Thresholds

Now that we've discussed some of the properties of the Big Three, let's briefly examine the issue of 'continua' versus 'thresholds' in mental illness. Recall that continua are things that exist as a smooth range, such as the temperature of the air, whereas thresholds are things that have an abrupt yes/no answer. Both phenomena definitely exist in the brain, and I think both can exist in cases of mental illness. My Case Study, for example, even contains examples of continua *with* thresholds: I responded to different doses of the drugs desipramine and Zyprexa in a continuous manner, with smoothly increasing responses to increases in dose, but when Zyprexa was increased beyond a threshold dose it caused the brain freeze. Just because the levels of the Big Three and their postsynaptic receptor populations are probably at least coarsely continuous within the population of all people, doesn't mean that during mental illness the brain can't exhibit thresholds. For example, consider these apparent thresholds: people with bipolar disorder may either exhibit mood cycling or not, and people with major depression may either exhibit early morning awakenings or not. Ser or nore circuitry dysfunction may also represent a threshold. In contrast, one study has shown that attention deficit hyperactivity disorder (ADHD), or at least hyperactivity among children, is a continuum, in which essentially *everyone* becomes less physically active when given ADHD stimulant drugs. In other words, there may not be a rigid threshold that distinguishes people with ADHD from those without ADHD. And as I'll discuss in Chapter 11, mood, or more generally expanded dysthymia, may be a continuum in which essentially everyone can be made better off or at least changed by Big Three altering drugs, as in The Adjustment. Finally, the current manner of diagnosing mental illness represents a threshold: one is said to either have or not have an illness.

CHAPTER 5

BIG THREE STRENGTH INTERACTIONS: THE TRIANGLE

Major Points

• The Big Three interact by affecting one another's strengths, illustrated by a simple diagram called 'The Triangle', where ser and nore form the base and dop forms the apex.

• The most important interaction is that ser and nore each strengthen dop, illustrating why certain antidepressants induce mania in people with bipolar disorder.

• Any drug that affects one of the Big Three is 'dirty' in that it also affects the other two.

Based on all the research to date, I believe that ser and nore (and possibly dop) interact by affecting the same circuitry. The Big Three may also interact in another way, by affecting each other's strengths directly, and this is of practical importance to treating mental illness. These strength interactions may take place in the brainstem (where the Big Three presynaptic neurons reside), or in the cerebral cortex (where the outputs of the Big Three presynaptic neurons are received by postsynaptic neurons), and may not involve the levels of the transmitters. There is growing evidence, particularly from studies of the rodent brain, that the Big Three affect each other's strengths, but the exact nature of these interactions is not clear and neither is their importance.

I refer to the Big Three strength interactions as 'The Triangle'

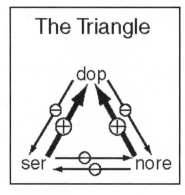

The Triangle

Figure 2

(see Figure 2), which is based on long-term interactions that take place over weeks or months (such as the effects of antidepressants) rather than short-term effects which take place over minutes, hours, or a few days, and have typically been observed in drug studies with animals. I do not mean to imply that the Big Three don't also interact with other neurotransmitter systems, but that The Triangle represents the principal strength interactions these three brain chemical systems have with each other.

Ser and nore form the base of The Triangle, partly because these two neurotransmitters are more similar in their brain distribution and function to one another than either is to dop. As we shall see, ser and nore appear to form a 'push-pull' pairing, since their effects on a number of characteristics and traits are directly opposed. Dop forms the apex of The Triangle. Here's the most important reason why: for individuals who suffer from bipolar disorder (manic-depressive illness), drugs that strengthen ser and drugs that strengthen nore both trigger mania. Mania is a condition in which an individual exhibits elevated mood, faster thinking, wildly ambitious (grandiose) ideas, hyperactivity, and often agitation. Since an increase in strength of either ser or nore can induce mania in a given bipolar individual, there seems to be some common factor that both of these neurotransmitters strengthen. That common factor is probably dop. Why's that? Firstly, the street drug cocaine, which strengthens dop, produces a 'high' that mimics mania, with the classic symptoms of incredible energy and feeling 'on top of the world'. Other drugs that strengthen dop, such as amphetamine and Ritalin, are capable of producing a similar high. Secondly, dop is distributed densely in the prefrontal region of the brain, which is thought to be involved in thinking, and therefore stronger dop may speed up thinking and possibly result in more grandiose thinking.

So dop appears to be capable of being strengthened by ser and nore in bipolar individuals. In addition, depressed individuals often report that their thoughts have slowed down, and instead of having grandiose ideas they tend to have very negative ideas. Administration of ser strengthening antidepressants and nore strengthening antidepressants often reverses these thought patterns, which is consistent with dop strengthening. And even in normal individuals, administration of an antidepressant such as Prozac, which strengthens ser, can speed up thought processes and boost self-esteem—both phenomena are described in *Listening to Prozac*—and there is evidence that Prozac strengthens dop in the rodent prefrontal cortex. The new attention deficit hyperactivity disorder (ADHD) drug, Strattera, which strengthens nore, has been shown to increase prefrontal levels of dop in rodents, and this has also been shown for reboxetine, an anti-depressant that strengthens nore.

These lines of evidence indicate that, in the human brain, dop is indeed strengthened when ser or nore is strengthened. In the basic diagram of The Triangle (see Figure 2), *thick plus arrows* pointing from ser and nore to dop describe this strong strengthening phenomenon. The *thin minus arrows* in the diagram indicate the opposite effect in all of the other interactions between the Big Three, weakening the neurotransmitters through what we'll call 'feedback inhibition'. This means that dop weakens both ser and nore, and that ser and nore weaken each other. As we shall see, feedback inhibition may explain several psychiatric phenomena, such as weak ser causing psychosis in some cases of schizophrenia and mania. In schizophrenia, typical antipsychotics such as Haldol and Thorazine may actually *strengthen* ser, and thereby terminate psychosis, through their known direct effect of weakening dop, since in The Triangle weakening dop strengthens ser because the feedback inhibition is diminished. Likewise, in most cases of mania, nore may have become super strong and thereby weakened ser, triggering psychosis. We will discuss schizophrenia and mania in more detail in Chapter 10.

The topic of Big Three strength interactions is related to the issue of how the brain maintains the strengths of each of the Big Three neurotransmitter systems in the first place, where I believe these systems are, for most people, quite constant throughout life. For example, when one of the Big Three is affected by an environmental factor such as a stressor and reaches a threshold strength, does the brain have a feedback mechanism that brings the neurotransmitter back to its normal strength? The brain does have presynaptic autoreceptors (see Figure 1) that sense the synaptic level of the transmitter and can then change the amount of transmitter that is released, but these mechanisms apparently aren't powerful enough to stop drugs from working—in the long term at least—or mental illness from developing. So the fact that psychiatric drugs usually work suggests that the brain does not have extremely robust long-term regulation of the Big Three strengths, and the fact that mental illnesses exist is consistent with this conclusion.

The current theory hypothesizes that the natural ser and nore systems (which are determined by genetics and past experiences) strengthen dop, as does strengthening ser and nore with drugs. Just because ser or nore strengthening drugs strengthen dop doesn't mean that the natural ser and nore systems must also strengthen dop, but this is an important assumption that has implications throughout this book. So under this premise and as described in The Triangle, the natural strength of dop should correlate with the sum of the natural ser and nore strengths. In other words, the stronger ser and nore are in a given person, the stronger her dop will also be.

If ser and nore really do strengthen dop, then most antidepressants are 'dirty' drugs in that their effects aren't restricted to a single neurotransmitter system. And if there are even more Big Three interactions as described in The Triangle, then any drug that affects one of the Big Three—and perhaps even a drug that affects only a single subtype of Big Three external receptors—is dirty. (Note: by 'external receptors' I mean receptors on the outer surface of the neuron; also known as 'extracellular receptors'.) Moreover, perhaps depressions really are always specific to one of the Big Three, but The Triangle explains why people may still respond to an antidepressant that changes the strength of any one of the Big Three.

CHAPTER 6

BIG THREE CIRCUITS

Major Points

• **How the Big Three act on brain circuits can be understood in terms of simple rules of logic.**

• **Ser and nore act on the same circuits and often have opposing effects, and dop may act on separate circuits.**

• **A single brain area may encode mood.**

• **The same circuits—essentially the whole brain—produce(s) both personality traits and mental illness.**

Now we'll discuss some aspects of the brain circuitry that the Big Three neurotransmitters act upon, focusing on the electrical properties of those circuits. We may not know how the circuits work in detail, but we can speculate as to how their responses are modulated by the Big Three. My working hypothesis is that ser and nore act upon the same postsynaptic neural circuits, having effects on those circuits that are distinct from the effects of dop, where the dop circuits may actually be separate. Most of the effects of ser and nore on those circuits are opposed: a push-pull relationship. This means that a drug that strengthens ser, for example, will in many ways have the opposite effect of a drug that strengthens nore.

Getting back to the circuitry, we have a pretty good idea of the Big Three presynaptic elements, namely the brainstem neurons, but the relevant postsynaptic circuits are much more poorly understood. Only a subset of a circuit's neurons may possess Big Three receptors, which makes the problem of identifying and understanding these circuits more difficult for neuroscientists.

Throughout this book we discuss the 'strengths' of Big Three neurotransmitter systems, where these strengths are directly related to the amount of electrical information that is transmitted through a circuit.

Levels of Scale

Let's continue our discussion of Big Three circuits by focusing at a microscopic scale, as there are undoubtedly many molecular factors that control the electrical properties of Big Three circuits. For example, there are many different proteins that control presynaptic neurotransmitter release, any one of which could affect the strength of the Big Three systems. Likewise, there are many different proteins involved in Big Three postsynaptic intracellular signaling cascades that may affect system strength, where such cascades are the principal response to the neurotransmitter binding to the receptor. In addition, Big Three external receptor populations may vary in density, structure, and sensitivity. Finally, the physical structure of the synapse can affect its sensitivity to the Big Three neurotransmitters, and thereby the strength of the system, as evidenced by the recent identification of synapse formation genes implicated in some cases of schizophrenia. This latter result provides concrete evidence that the *level* of ser alone may not explain the illness in some people, but nonetheless in these cases the illness could still probably be treated by resetting or strengthening ser with drugs (see Chapter 10).

What does all of this complexity at a molecular scale mean for our purposes? Two things: 1) future drugs may be able to adjust Big Three strengths in novel ways by affecting these molecular properties and thereby improving mental health treatment; 2) many, many genes affect Big Three strengths, which may bode poorly for applying the findings of ongoing genetic studies to improve mental health treatment, at least in the near future.

We can continue our discussion of circuitry at a slightly larger scale. At the level of the single neuron, there are different types of neurons with different physical structures and functional properties; on a slightly larger scale there are different layers of interconnected neurons within a cortical area. In mammals, most cortical areas consist of six principal layers, and each layer can consist of multiple sublayers; next there are different systems of interconnected cortical areas, such as the 30+ areas constituting a single sensory channel such as vision; and finally there are whole brain networks that provide integration of multiple cortical systems, as in the neural integrator hypothesis or the binding problem, both mentioned earlier.

When scientists come to understand these larger-scale brain properties better, what would this mean for our purposes? Two things: 1) These aspects of the circuitry need to be considered during brain imaging studies of mental illness, such as those using PET and MRI scans. For example, if multiple brain areas are deactivated by a particular mental illness, perhaps the average decrease in metabolic activity in each brain area correlates with the severity of the illness, or perhaps there is a more complex mathematical interaction between the separate brain areas that indicates the severity. 2) To fully understand how a Big Three drug affects the brain, we need to know its overall effect on these large-scale circuits, and in humans this would mean monitoring those effects with brain imaging methods in a very precise manner.

Effects of Drugs

Let's now take a closer look at the effects of drugs on Big Three circuits. Just because there may be single, systemic Big Three levels throughout the brain, doesn't mean drugs can't activate subsets of the circuits by functioning as activators or deactivators for particular receptor subtypes, since many such subtypes exist. For example, there are a wide variety of ser receptor subtypes, such as the 5HT_2A receptor, and subtype specific drugs exist that may produce more specific perceptual effects than level altering drugs such as Prozac. And just because there may be one systemic level for each of the Big Three doesn't mean that level has uniform effects on all circuits—the circuitry in different brains and different parts of a single brain may differ dramatically in the way in which it interacts with the transmitter, not necessarily limited to differences in sensitivity to that transmitter.

If the postsynaptic circuitry changes strength in response to a greater or lesser level of ser or nore produced by a Big Three drug, 'thinking' that this is the genetic level of ser or nore, then why doesn't the brain have less limited plasticity for the adjustment of ser or nore in a given person (it didn't in My Case Study, for example, due to the brain freeze)? In other words, the brain may only be capable of adjusting to quite limited Big Three strength changes caused by drugs, though these changes can nonetheless be very beneficial to a given person, as in My Case Study.

Concerning the brain basis of responses to Big Three drugs, it could be that Big Three external receptors upregulate or downregulate on a very fast timescale—changing their numbers or sensitivity on a daily basis or even within minutes—but it might be dangerously unstable for the brain to operate this way, and therefore unlikely that it evolved to do so.

The Big Three may only be the principal neurotransmitters at the initial stage or stages of the postsynaptic circuitry, whereas other transmitters, such as glutamate (the brain's principal excitatory transmitter) or GABA (the brain's principal inhibitory transmitter), may affect later stages. Therefore, maybe the Big Three merely provide one of many ways to adjust such circuitry with drugs. So perhaps the Big Three circuits can be adjusted more dramatically by multiple adjustments within the pathway of each circuit, by using additional drugs with non-Big Three mechanisms. In other words, if there are multiple steps in a pathway, maybe there is a limit to how much each step can be adjusted, and this might be capitalized upon by off-label drugs (which are prescribed for non-psychiatric treatments, such as arthritis) or future drugs which, when used in conjunction with existing drugs, might improve mental health treatment substantially.

Circuit Modulation

How do the Big Three actually modulate the electrical properties of their circuits? As stated previously, the simplest form of circuit modulation by the Big Three is activation or inactivation. Another type of modulation is the more complex circuit transformation, changing its functional properties, rather than simply turning the circuit further on or off. Such modulation may take place in a continuous manner, thresholded manner, or both. And a circuit may have a baseline condition that would exist even in the absence of the Big Three: turned on, turned off, transformed, dysfunctional, or more than one effect. An important point is that in a given individual, circuits may be largely turned on or off in the absence of overt, or at least pronounced, mood disorder or other mental illness, as in expanded dysthymia (see Chapter 11)—emotion could be one such circuit, though there are probably different circuits for different emotions.

What do the Big Three systems tell us about the logic of circuit modulation, as in the type of reasoning and componentry an engineer might use to build an electrical circuit? We can imagine a large number of complex interactions that these transmitters might have with their circuitry, or that might occur downstream within those circuits, but let's consider two simple cases: AND and OR, where I will define the two as mutually exclusive. Other possibilities: NOT, IF THEN, or more complex operators. AND means that each of the Big

Three, or at least both ser and nore, is required for proper circuit functioning, whereas OR means that any one of the Big Three can independently affect the circuit in a similar manner. I think that AND is the correct model. For example, the absence of depression may require ser AND nore to both be at mid-range, non-dysfunctional strengths. More generally, the Big Three systems may all need to be completely intact for optimal mental health, also an AND. However, psychiatrists often treat depression as an OR for ser and nore, believing that drugs that strengthen ser, nore, or both will all be similarly effective, though I don't think this is true. Regardless of whether the Big Three circuits are affected in an AND or an OR manner, only one of the Big Three systems may be awry in a particular case of mental illness.

Mood Circuits

Where in the brain are the Big Three mood circuits? The relatively new deep brain stimulation technique, which produces a potent antidepressant effect in depressed patients by activating particular brain areas (such as area 25) with a surgically implanted electrode, provides clues, as do brain imaging studies of depressed and bipolar persons. I think of mood as probably encoded by an area or areas in either prefrontal cortex, limbic cortex, or both. And though sensory cortical systems consist of multiple brain areas, there may be a single cortical area that encodes mood because it may not require as much information processing as a sensory system.

Personality Traits and Mental Illness

I will argue that the same circuits—essentially the whole brain—produce(s) personality traits and mental illness, though this is a big leap considering that these circuits could be separate and independent. But if they are one and the same, is everyone's brain circuitry essentially the same, except for differences in the Big Three among different people? Probably not. Instead, I think there are hardwired, permanent, largely genetic differences in circuitry between individuals, including general, consistent differences between men and women, as well as Big Three strength differences. Moreover, maybe some types or at least cases of mental illness or personality traits are hardwired into the brain—perhaps including neuronal damage from mental illness, such as brain atrophy in some cases of long-term schizophrenia—and can be corrected only to a limited extent, or not at all, by drugs.

The mental illnesses—and personality traits—also tend to blend into one another among different people, which probably mirrors activation of the Big Three circuits, and all people do not experience the 'same' illness in the same way. Such coexistence of multiple mental illnesses (such as schizophrenia and obsessive-compulsive disorder (OCD), or bipolar disorder and eating disorders) in people is consistent with a single level of each of the Big Three throughout the brain affecting multiple mental illness producing circuits. It could also be caused by functional overlap in the circuits themselves, or individual circuits may be common to multiple illnesses. Indeed, different mental illnesses in the same person would co-occur 100% of the time if they were produced by the same circuit.

CHAPTER 7

BIG THREE FUNCTIONS

Major Points

• **The Big Three affect a large number of traits in addition to mood, both in the presence and in the absence of mental illness, and thereby have a profound influence on both personality and mental illness.**

• **Ser and nore together may form a cognitive-sensory-emotional filter, with a high ser/nore ratio deadening these entities.**

• **Strong nore may be associated with physical endurance, cancer, and homosexuality.**

Now we'll discuss some of the traits that the Big Three may affect, including: thought, sensation, emotion, mood, stress tolerance, drive states (such as hunger and thirst), sleep, movement, learning and memory, disease, and gender differences/sexual preference. I hypothesize that each of these traits is affected by the Big Three both in the presence and in the absence of overt mental illness. In this section we'll focus on the effects of the Big Three in the absence of overt mental illness, and in Chapter 10 we'll discuss the relationship between the Big Three and specific mental illnesses. By having all of these functions, the Big Three have a profound influence on both personality and mental illness, in essence because these functions, or disturbances of them, produce personality and mental illness, and thereby drastically affect our experience of the world and quality of life. I think these traits also tend to correlate in a given person, consistent with the existence of the neural integrator or at least common Big Three input to various circuits. The bottom line is that the Big Three do a lot more than just affect mood. And keep in mind that a given person with weak ser, for example, may only exhibit a subset of the traits associated with weak ser that I have described below.

Thought

Thought is at least principally a prefrontal cortical phenomenon, and this region of the brain receives strong Big Three input, particularly from dop. The Big Three affect both the rate and subject matter of thought—cocaine strengthens dop strongly and causes both faster and more grandiose thinking, as well as paranoia. Ser and nore may only affect the subject matter of thought, with ser (and possibly nore) serving to filter out minor details, consistent with their roles in dominance discussed in Chapter 13. Thereby, strong ser (and possibly strong nore) produce instinctive intelligence, whereas weak ser produces technical intelligence. In other words, people with strong ser tend to think about the most salient phenomena, or the 'big picture', whereas people with weak ser tend to think about fine details. There are, however, exceptions to this simple model.

Self-esteem is at least partially a type of thought, and is also related to mood. As described in *Listening to Prozac*, ser plays an important role here, and its strength may be proportional to self-esteem. Dop strength may also be proportional to self-esteem; so self-esteem should correlate with the sum of ser and dop strength, though this is not to say that Big Three strengths are the only factors that contribute to self-esteem, to the exclusion of life experiences.

Speech is a reflection of thought, and difficulty articulating speech may represent a state of hypofrontality, discussed in Chapter 10. Obsessive thinking, as in obsessive-compulsive disorder (OCD), is related to activation of subcortical basal ganglia circuits (which are brain areas that affect movement and cognition) that can be affected by the Big Three (most well established for ser strengthening drugs).

Sensation

Sensation is defined here in the traditional manner, namely as consisting of the five basic senses: vision, hearing, taste, smell, and touch. According to My Case Study, ser deadens the senses and nore heightens the senses. In addition, depression or simply expanded dysthymia (discussed in Chapter 11) also deadens, and very likely at least transforms, the senses. So with equal amounts of dysthymia, higher nore/ser ratio people should have more acute senses than lower ratio people. In summary, both expanded dysthymia and the ser/nore ratio affect sensation.

Additional evidence that ser and nore affect sensation: 1) the street drug LSD affects sensation and acts on ser receptors, and 2) ser and nore brainstem neurons connect to sensory cortex. Furthermore, my perception of people—with women looking more attractive— was affected by ser altering drugs and nore altering drugs, consistent with sensory perception not being an objective, point-for-point representation of the world.

Since someone with a high ser/nore ratio has strongly deadened senses, the world may seem to be 'held at arm's length', whereas for someone with a low such ratio, the world may seem to be 'up in one's face'. Such sensory filtering may partially explain why strong ser can produce dominance.

The bottom line is that sensory acuity, like emotional responsiveness and characteristic thought patterns, is part of personality (a trait). For example, sharper senses may lead to a greater sense of aesthetics. Psychophysical studies, which are psychological experiments aimed at measuring properties of sensory perception, have shown that people perform differently on measures of sensory acuity. The current theory suggests that women tend to have sharper senses than men due to an average ser/nore ratio difference—though this difference may be counteracted if women tend to exhibit depression or expanded dysthymia more commonly than men—including a more refined sense of smell than men, which has been demonstrated experimentally.

Emotion

Combining the hypotheses about ser and nore affecting thought and sensation, ser and nore may together form a cognitive-sensory-emotional filter, with a high ser/nore ratio producing deadening of these entities and a low ser/nore ratio producing heightening, though this idea may not apply to those exhibiting nore dominance (see Chapter 13). By cognitive deadening, I mean that the person tends to think about the most important phenomena, not that her rate of thinking is slowed. By sensory deadening, I mean that her senses are less acute. By emotional deadening, I mean that the intensity of her emotions is diminished. If ser and nore form such a filter, ser and nore may produce alteration of thoughts, senses, and emotions in addition to affecting the properties mentioned above.

The Big Three may also affect the ability to experience pleasure. For example, psychiatrist Peter Kramer reports in *Listening to Prozac* that some of his patients who took Prozac, a ser strengthening drug, had greater ability to experience pleasure. More generally, expanded dysthymia, which involves non-optimal Big Three strengths, diminishes the ability to experience pleasure.

One's general level of interest in things is probably mediated emotionally. Ser may universally deaden interest, by deadening interest in all things, and nore may universally heighten interest, which is related to instinctive and technical intelligence. One could also hypothesize that expanded dysthymia (which is characterized by non-optimal strengths of ser and/or nore) deadens interest, and euthymia (which is characterized by optimal, mid-range strengths of ser and nore) heightens it. So both factors probably contribute to level of interest. Moreover, dominance itself may affect general level of interest by diminishing it.

Strong ser encodes compassion (as in Peter Kramer's observations), strong nore may encode empathy and jealousy, and, most importantly, having optimal strengths of ser and nore—lack of expanded dysthymia—produces most of the positive emotions. In other words, a dysthymic strong ser/weak nore person should not have the same emotional profile as an equally dysthymic strong nore/weak ser person. In addition, weakening nore may produce emotional stabilization, since nore may play a general role in intensifying emotions, and such stabilization may be beneficial if the individual is overly sensitive emotionally. Finally, a study of the nore weakening beta blocking drug propranolol indicates that nore plays a role in allowing a person to recognize facial expressions of sadness in others.

Mood

Mood can be thought of as a baseline state of how one feels, whereas emotions are alterations produced by stimuli, such as thoughts or sensations, and are superimposed upon mood. I think the Big Three must be at mid-range strengths to produce optimal, constant mood. An important point is that the brain can be 'turned off' by Big Three strength abnormalities while mood is still within the normal range or even high (hypomanic). For example, people with expanded dysthymia, which is characterized by non-optimal Big Three strengths, may not report feeling sad, but normal positive reaction to external events is muffled or even completely absent due to a constant, lower than optimal mood.

Stress Tolerance

If ser and nore have opposite effects on stress tolerance—with ser increasing it and nore decreasing it—this is consistent with ser dominance but may not apply to individuals exhibiting nore dominance. Nonetheless, drugs that strengthen ser, such as Prozac, can increase stress tolerance and decrease anxiety, and drugs that strengthen nore, such as yohimbine, can decrease stress tolerance and heighten anxiety. Dop may also increase stress tolerance, consistent with its role in dominance.

Drive States

Drive states such as hunger, thirst, and libido are also affected by the Big Three, including during mental illness. These entities can be either too strong or too weak when the Big Three are at non-optimal strengths, and this may partially explain why so many people have weight problems, since non-optimal strengths are so common (see Chapter 11). Ser boosting drugs such as the SRIs can deaden the libido, though they can also restore it by treating depression or expanded dysthymia.

Sleep

One of the functions of sleep may be to regulate the *levels* of the Big Three. This is a chicken and egg issue because sleep may regulate the Big Three levels and the Big Three levels may in turn regulate sleep. During waking, the brainstem ser and nore neurons fire action potentials—and thereby release neurotransmitter—in response to stimuli and also at a baseline level, fire more slowly during NREM (non-rapid eye movement) sleep, and don't fire at all during REM sleep. Therefore, as stated in Chapter 4, ser and nore synaptic levels build as the day wears on and are reabsorbed during sleep. Perhaps when a minimal ser or nore level is achieved during sleep reabsorption, one wakes up, or when there's too much of these transmitters one sleeps too much. And in explaining the effects of the Big Three on sleep, it may be important to distinguish between NREM and REM sleep, as their ratio of duration and absolute amounts are affected in depression, for example, and sleep disturbance can occur in mental illnesses other than depression and bipolar disorder. The conservative conclusion at this point is that the Big Three affect sleep but the precise nature of the effect has yet to be determined. In addition, the neurotransmitter acetylcholine clearly plays a role in sleep.

The point is that sleep is a largely objective measure of mental illness and possibly the functioning of the Big Three, though no simple relationship between the Big Three and sleep may exist that is consistent across all individuals. So abnormal sleep may be neither necessary nor sufficient for mental illness, but nonetheless may provide objective, additional evidence that it exists in a given case.

Movement

There is no reason why the Big Three can't affect movement, since they are present in the motor cortex, cerebellum, and spinal cord (and for nore, the heart), and these parts of the central nervous system are intimately involved in generating movement. For example, there is potentially a relationship between movement and dominance, since swift, powerful movements and high energy may aid in achieving and maintaining dominance, and dominance itself may be strongly affected by the Big Three (see Chapter 13).

There may also be a relationship between strong nore and physical endurance, since endurance athletes, such as marathon runners and cyclists (example: Lance Armstrong), tend to have the personality traits (see Chapter 12) of super strong nore. And beta blockers, which weaken nore, can reduce endurance. If strong nore really does produce improved endurance, surely it doesn't do so solely by affecting the motor cortex—the mechanism may be mediated by connections with the heart, spinal cord, or other aspects of the peripheral nervous system. So perhaps ser and dop enhance explosive movements, whereas nore enhances sustained movements.

If the Big Three affect aspects of motor performance, then do they also affect taste preference, and therefore preference for intake of certain types of food? Food preference may be strongly linked to movement, and may serve to further enhance the biases that the Big Three already place on characteristics of movement. Ser and dop may increase a preference for foods that enhance explosive movements (such as simple carbohydrates), and nore may increase a preference for foods that enhance sustained movements (such as vegetables). So due to the potential role of the Big Three in biasing movement, Big Three altering drugs may be athletically performance enhancing, or at least altering, tools.

Learning and Memory

The Big Three very likely affect learning and memory, including but not necessarily limited to their effects on thought patterns, described earlier in this chapter. For example, abnormally low strengths of the Big Three may cause hypofrontality—which is poor attention and poor memory due to underfunctioning of prefrontal cortex—or instead high strengths may produce normal to supranormal prefrontal functional enhancement. During mental illness, learning and memory are almost always perturbed, usually in a negative manner, as was the case in My Case Study. However, cognitive functions such as learning and memory have been more closely associated with another modulatory neurotransmitter, acetylcholine.

Disease

If Big Three strength abnormalities or dysfunction cause diseases in addition to mental illnesses, it could be because of the mental illnesses they produce, or because of the abnormal strengths or dysfunction themselves, independent of mental illness. In other words, the established association of heart disease being worsened by depression may be due to abnormal Big Three strengths and not the depression. This principle may be relevant for Parkinson's disease and dop, or Alzheimer's disease and acetylcholine, where these two transmitter systems are closely associated with these two respective diseases.

In either case, I think asthma and some types of cancer are associated with strong nore, due to the personality traits of a number of people I have either known or known about who had these diseases. Likewise, mitral valve prolapse—a heart abnormality—is associated with autonomic (i.e., the part of the nervous system that regulates involuntary action, and uses nore as a signaling molecule) hypersensitivity, consistent with a strong systemic nore basis. Perhaps these diseases could be prevented or, in the case of asthma, treated with drugs that weaken nore, such as clonidine.

Certain types of epilepsy may be associated with Big Three strength abnormalities, since Big Three drugs, such as certain antidepressants, can trigger seizures. Likewise, migraine headaches may be caused by weak ser and/or strong nore, since drugs that strengthen ser and drugs that weaken nore can provide effective treatment.

Gender Differences and Sexual Preference
I think men tend, on average, to be slightly stronger in ser and slightly weaker in nore than women, though there seems to be a huge amount of overlap between the two sexes in these two strengths. There are now PET brain imaging data that indicate that men, on average, tend to synthesize about 50% more ser than women. This putative ser strength difference may at least partially explain the higher reported rates of depression in women. Based on this hypothesis, I initially thought that the ser and nore systems form the basis of masculinity and femininity, or at least heterosexuality and homosexuality— namely that heterosexual men tend to be strong in ser, weak in nore, whereas homosexual men tend to be strong in nore, weak in ser. And heterosexual women tend to be strong in nore, weak in ser, whereas

homosexual women tend to be strong in ser, weak in nore. This is probably an oversimplification, particularly since many bisexual or homosexual women have the personality traits of super strong nore— examples: Ellen DeGeneres, Anne Heche, Martina Navratilova. However, perhaps all male bisexuals and homosexuals have strong nore (as may effeminate men), as if strong nore is necessary but not sufficient for male homosexuality. This sort of reasoning leads to the conclusion that a sexual ambiguity/homosexuality circuit exists in certain brains, the activation of which requires strong nore. So maybe one factor that can affect masculinity or femininity is ser and nore strengths, and drugs that affect ser or nore may subtly affect sexual preference. Mania and depression, which probably involve Big Three abnormalities, certainly can affect sexual potency, though not necessarily sexual preference.

One important component of sexuality is pattern recognition circuitry for responding to the opposite sex, including visual (face/body cues) and other sensory cues. The greater the optimality of ser and nore, as in My Case Study, the greater the activation of this circuitry, resulting in greater perceived prominence of these cues. Remember, in My Case Study, when ser and nore were adjusted with drugs closer to mid-range strengths, women actually *looked* more attractive, probably because this circuitry was more activated. Mental illnesses, including but not limited to bipolar disorder and major depression, may also affect this circuitry.

I think women tend to experience stronger emotions than men, even when individuals from the two sexes have the same underlying Big Three strengths. So ser and nore differences probably don't explain all of the differences between the male and female brains, including potentially many hardwired circuitry differences. Maybe the same circuit that produces homosexuality affects the emotions, or these circuits correlate in activation. So the male and female Big Three emotion circuits may be a lot different from one another, but do the male and female brains differ in other traits listed here as Big Three functions, other than sensory acuity which I discussed earlier?

Miscellaneous Traits

Now I'll touch upon a few other traits that may be affected by the Big Three. Coldness perception is defined here as the subjective feeling of how cold it is, and it may be affected by the Big Three. Ser may increase coldness sensitivity (at least it did for me, while I was hypomanic on Zoloft, though for some people it may decrease sensitivity), nore may decrease coldness sensitivity (at least it does anecdotally in some cases of mania), and dop may have no effect on coldness sensitivity. Ser (and nore, dop) may also affect the traits explored in Peter Kramer's *Listening to Prozac*: compulsiveness, rejection sensitivity, and risk taking.

There's an established link between weak ser and violence. Maybe some weak ser individuals tend to perceive other people as threatening, and this makes violence more likely; or perhaps their potentially low, irritable mood plays a role. Nonetheless, it is probably incorrect to say that weak ser is necessary but not sufficient for violence, since other Big Three strength arrays can probably also produce violence—it's more accurate to say that weak ser interacting with particular hardwired circuitry may make violence more likely. So prisons may in some ways be the modern vestiges of the state mental hospitals so abundant in the United States prior to the 1950s.

CHAPTER 8

THE ADJUSTMENT

Major Points

• The Adjustment is a method for using existing pharmaceutical drugs to tweak a person's Big Three strengths closer to optimal, mid-range values (i.e., not too strong or too weak). Doing so not only treats nearly every type of mental illness but also may improve quality of life for over 50% of the population.

• The Adjustment affects many more traits than just mood, though mood is an important trait that is affected.

• To perform The Adjustment properly in a given person, two drugs are often needed to tweak ser and nore independently, often in opposite strength directions.

• Most people, whether they suffer from a mental illness or not, have weak ser and/or strong nore.

• If the field of psychiatry were to implement The Adjustment in nearly every person seeking mental health treatment, that treatment would be vastly improved.

The Adjustment is a method whereby existing pharmaceutical drugs are used to tweak the strengths of ser and nore (and possibly dop) closer to optimal, mid-range values. The current theory hypothesizes that doing so not only treats nearly every type of overt mental illness, but also may improve quality of life, possibly dramatically, for many people (expanded dysthymics, who may constitute over 50% of the population—more on this subject in Chapter 11) who are considered normal. As we have been discussing, performing The Adjustment—a type of Big Three strength modification—affects many more traits than just mood, though mood is an important trait that is affected. An adjustment in the right direction should make people better (higher self-reported quality of life, possibly also apparent to an outside observer), and an adjustment in the wrong direction should make people worse. Adjusting dop is a secondary, less important adjustment. I don't see strong dop as pathological, unless it's so strong that it underlies mania/marked hypomania and mood cycling. However, weak dop, which may be associated with underfunctioning of the frontal lobes resulting in diminished thinking, may be pathological. As we'll discuss in the next chapter, all six categories of drugs for The Adjustment exist and are FDA approved in the United States: 1) drugs that strengthen ser, 2) drugs that weaken ser (many of which also weaken dop), 3) drugs that strengthen nore, 4) drugs that weaken nore, 5) drugs that strengthen dop, and 6) drugs that weaken dop (most of which also weaken ser).

For many people The Adjustment will involve polytherapy—which is the use of more than one drug at a time—since both ser and nore (and even dop) may have to be adjusted, possibly in opposite strength directions. In such a case, adjusting both ser and nore up or down can produce a synergistic effect that may be different not only in magnitude, but also in character, than adjusting either one alone, in that the net effect is different than the sum of its parts, and this is not due to interactions in metabolizing the drugs.

For example, if a person has weak ser and strong nore, then, in order to perform The Adjustment, one drug will be needed to strengthen ser and another drug will be needed to weaken nore. If you think you may have bipolar disorder, definitely start the nore or ser weakening drug first, because a nore or ser strengthening drug can trigger mania or hypomania in bipolars, which is not a good thing, and it is controversial whether to use such a strengthening drug at all in bipolar disorder. Even if you don't have bipolar disorder, I don't recommend starting both drugs at the same time, mainly because it will be hard to tell which drug is doing what, including the possible side effects, or whether both drugs are even necessary. Start one first, such as the nore weakener clonidine (class of drugs: alpha 2 adrenergic agonists), assessing whether it has a positive effect on quality of life, and if so wait a month or so to let it take full effect. The dose of the drug can also be tweaked, and you should wait a month or so for full effect, though too high a dose may be unpleasant and not recommended. If, on the other hand, there is no response at all to this first drug, then try another drug from the same class, such as the nore weakener guanfacine. If the drug has a negative effect on quality of life, then perhaps that drug and that class of drugs is not recommended for you. After you and your doctor have decided what to do with the first type of drug, including whether to even take it, then the second type of drug can be added in a similar manner.

Based on people's personality traits, all forms of adjustments may be needed for real people: all combinations of weak, medium (mid-range), and strong for each of the Big Three may exist in the population, except both strong ser and strong nore. It's as if there is a practical limit to the sum of ser and nore strength in the brain. Moreover, the most common pair of strengths is weak ser and/or strong nore.

I'm not arguing that Big Three adjustments are the only neuro-chemical adjustments that affect quality of life, just that they are adjustments that will affect everyone or nearly everyone in principle with the existing drugs—or with potential new drugs with similar or dissimilar Big Three mechanisms. It should also be noted that the range of change of Big Three strengths that the current drugs can produce is probably much smaller than the range of genetic differences of Big Three strengths in the population, but large enough to cause a profound change in quality of life in at least some people. Similarly, the individuals with the greatest potential response to The Adjustment are probably those with the least optimal ser and nore strengths.

100% of people would respond to a Big Three strength adjustment, but at this time probably not everyone can have these strengths adjusted with the existing drugs. For example, in a given person the existing drugs may not bind properly to her particular Big Three receptors. It's also possible that some people could never have their strengths adjusted by *any* future drug, though this percentage is probably close to zero if not zero.

How could psychiatrists go about implementing The Adjustment most effectively in a given person? Well, blood levels of the Big Three, which researchers have been measuring for many years, if they indeed reflect brain strengths, would be useful in deciding how to adjust a person as well as provide monitoring of the effects of The Adjustment. Brain imaging techniques, such as PET and MRI scans, may also indicate how to adjust a given person as well as provide monitoring of the effects of The Adjustment. And assessing Big Three personality traits, if this can be done accurately and consistently, may also be useful for implementing and monitoring The Adjustment.

The Adjustment may be the neurochemical basis for making some depressed people 'better than well', as in Peter Kramer's patients in *Listening to Prozac*—in other words, his patients had weak ser, and possibly weak dop. However, the potential benefits of the technique must be weighed against the risk of causing a 3+ year brain freeze like I accidentally suffered while The Adjustment was being performed on me (see My Case Study—Chapter 2). Other people besides myself have probably unwittingly experienced the full adjustment while being treated for psychiatric and non-psychiatric conditions simultaneously, since many of the relevant drugs have non-psychiatric uses. The Adjustment may also be a way to adjust the neural integrator, if the integrator exists (see Chapter 2).

A common misconception about antidepressants—a subset of The Adjustment drugs—is that they only deaden the emotions. When used properly, I believe they can heighten emotions, and in general improve quality of life. And maybe only drugs that weaken ser and/or nore (or only those that deactivate ser and/or nore postsynaptic receptors, such as Zyprexa) can cause the brain freeze, whereas drugs that strengthen ser and/or nore cannot. More generally, the brain freeze may occur when the strengths of ser and nore are adjusted in opposite directions—either closer to or farther away from optimal, mid-range strengths—and the magnitude of such an adjustment exceeds some limit. Nevertheless, the benefits to those who are suffering from long-term mental illness certainly make it worth their while to work with a health care professional to implement, at the very least, some component of The Adjustment.

CHAPTER 9

EFFECTS OF DRUGS

Major Points

• There already exist the six categories of FDA approved drugs to strengthen or weaken each of the Big Three, and thereby perform The Adjustment.

• The proposed nore weakening drugs are not yet widely used by psychiatrists and their use could result in landmark improvements in treatment.

• The brain mechanism of the hallucinogenic street drug LSD is relevant to understanding psychotic brain states, such as those found in schizophrenia.

The existing drugs should allow us to perform The Adjustment, and thereby for better or worse, allow us in part to undo what genetics and stress have done. Drugs may eventually, and to some extent probably already do, allow us to 'access' the Big Three circuitry at different points in each pathway, affecting personality traits as well as affecting mental illness characteristics. A given Big Three drug may treat more than one type of mental illness, just as it may affect many personality traits.

While we may not know the possibly harmful long-term effects of taking psychiatric drugs, we also don't know the possibly harmful effects of having abnormal Big Three systems or mental illnesses themselves, such as potential brain damage. As mentioned in Chapter 7, there's already a known association between depression exacerbating heart disease, and Big Three abnormalities may also be associated with other diseases.

Drugs that act on the ser and nore systems are not physically addictive in the conventional sense because they do not produce physical craving. On the other hand, such drugs can produce withdrawal effects, though these tend to be quite mild. Drugs that act directly on the dop system, such as cocaine and crystal methamphetamine, are physically addictive, and part of their addictiveness may derive from their ability to produce an immediate 'high'. The dop D2 receptor is thought to be the principal brain receptor acted upon either directly (via boosting the level of dop), as in cocaine and crystal meth, or indirectly as in alcohol or even food itself, which is relevant to eating disorders. The reason the D2 receptor is implicated in these disorders is because it plays an important role in the brain's normal reward system, in that stimulation of this receptor makes the person temporarily feel good.

Most psychiatric drugs with known mechanisms of action affect the Big Three, and many of the drugs with unknown mechanisms may also do so indirectly, or at least act on the same circuits. Ideally we would use ser, nore, or dop specific drugs for The Adjustment, and ideally these drugs would have no or minimal metabolic interaction, which means that one drug would not interfere with the rate at which the body breaks down and eliminates another drug. At the one extreme there are receptor subtype specific drugs (or even potentially more specific intracellular drugs), whereas at the other extreme are drugs that strengthen or weaken—or activate or deactivate multiple receptors of—more than one Big Three neurotransmitter system. The latter type of drugs casts a broader net, though simultaneously using several drugs of the former type would be more precise for implementing The Adjustment in a given person.

A premise of the current theory is that there is no difference between altering the strengths of the Big Three with a drug and altering the strengths based on the natural functioning of the brain, which is mainly produced by genetics and also by environmental inputs such as stressors. For example, is antidepressant induced mania somehow different than mania that occurs naturally? Or is antidepressant induced wellness somehow different than normal, natural mood? The assumption here is that the drugs can produce the same effects as natural Big Three strengths.

Reversibility of effect, namely that the effects of a given drug will go away once it is discontinued—though there still are potential withdrawal effects—is an important consideration in using psychiatric drugs. This usually applies to all currently used drugs except the typical antipsychotics, which can cause tardive dyskinesia, a potentially irreversible movement disorder. Very rare irreversible effects may take place with other drugs as well, such as lithium damaging the kidneys. Another type of reversible effect is side effects that go away after taking a drug for some time. On the other hand, ECT and antidepressants may sometimes produce irreversible positive effects, such as stopping major depression. So an individual doesn't always return to the prior, baseline unmedicated state after the drugs are withdrawn.

Flux is a term I use for temporary mild depression that a person can experience while the Big Three are being adjusted with drugs. Such drug adjustments can make a person transiently worse before eventually making them better. Rapidly (daily, weekly, or even monthly) changing types of drugs and/or their dosages may produce a continuous state of flux, as in My Case Study.

Due to postsynaptic saturation discussed in Chapter 4, drugs that *strengthen* ser and/or nore shouldn't immediately have a perceptible effect, though dop drugs do. Therefore, in the treatment of mental illness, the time of day in taking ser/nore drugs should be irrelevant, except for possible side effects (unless, for some reason, the postsynaptic receptors are not saturated). In contrast, Big Three *weakening* drugs should have an immediately perceptible effect, if, in the case of ser and nore, the level of weakening exceeds the safety factor. In practice, though, most drugs that weaken ser and/or nore still take two weeks to kick in because of the safety factor. However, it has already been demonstrated that propranolol, a nore weakening drug, *immediately* affects recognition of sad facial expressions.

The current psychiatric drugs, except for perhaps the SRIs, aren't exactly 'recreational drugs' due to significant potential side effects, including withdrawal effects. And even the SRIs can have serious side effects. There may be at least three types of side effects for a Big Three drug that is intended to be transmitter specific: 1) binding to non-Big Three receptors, 2) producing a physiologically abnormal response within the targeted transmitter system (example: SRIs causing agitation), 3) producing a physiologically normal response within the targeted transmitter system that is unwanted (example: SRIs causing anorgasmia). For 3), the sexual side effects of ser strengthening antidepressants, such as Prozac, may actually be direct consequences of strengthening ser.

The brain doesn't seem to adapt or return to baseline in response to changes in Big Three strengths caused by continuously taken drug dosages, but in the rest of the body, like the gut or the heart, there may be adaptation. For example, the SRIs often upset the gut for a few weeks while they are kicking in, but then the gut adapts and returns to normal. Maybe people who claim to have *brain* adaptation during the treatment of mental illness are softly bipolar, have a recurrent or periodic illness such as unipolar depression, or have a seasonal pattern to their illness. If there really is brain adaptation in some cases, how common is it? Does it just occur in certain subpopulations of patients or with certain drugs? Can it be 'fooled' by introducing a different drug from the same class, a drug from another class, or the same drug at a later time?

Within a class of drugs (say SRIs), when there's non-response to one drug and response to another in a given person, this probably implies lack of binding to the particular receptor or receptors for the non-responding drug. (Another possibility is that the drug wasn't absorbed properly.) In other words, when a level boosting antidepressant, or any other Big Three receptor-based drug, doesn't work, it is usually because the key doesn't fit the lock on a molecular scale, in terms of the drug/receptor interaction. However, just because a drug binds to a receptor doesn't mean it will produce the intended effect. So the first place to look for variability in the effects of specific receptor-based drugs among different people is in the actual binding to those receptors. One future improvement for psychiatry would be understanding the three-dimensional structures of different alleles (variants of a gene) of the receptors and thereby figuring out how well the drugs bind, or at least seeing how alleles correlate with different Big Three traits and mental illnesses, as well as whether certain alleles predict response to certain Big Three drugs. Finally, from a pharmacological perspective, why does everyone seem to respond to street drugs, such as cocaine, LSD, and marijuana and not to antidepressants and other psychiatric drugs?

Drugs that bind directly to specific postsynaptic receptors are in principle more specific in their effects than drugs that simply raise or lower the level of the transmitter, since changing the level can affect a wide array of receptors. Drugs that directly enter the postsynaptic neurons in order to achieve their effects—which I call intracellular drugs—may also activate the brain circuitry in a very specific manner. Creating more drugs with more specific effects may lead to improved treatment of mental illness.

Scientists are already able to measure Big Three levels in the blood, urine, and cerebrospinal fluid (CSF). Measuring Big Three responses to a transmitter level altering drug such as an antidepressant, coupled with blood measurement of the drug level itself, may provide useful information about a person's response to the drug. And to best implement The Adjustment, one could first perform baseline blood measurement of the levels of the Big Three, which would tell one which type of drug to use if indeed blood measures correlate with brain strengths.

There's already a large body of evidence showing that anti-depressants do a lot more than just affect mood. The greatest amount of evidence exists for SRIs, affecting traits related to dominance, for example. Antidepressants also seem to affect the rate and subject matter of thought in everyone, not just bipolar or depressed persons.

Are some antidepressants more effective than others at treating depression? Conventional wisdom is that every existing anti-depressant provides at least some relief to about 60-80% of depressed people, but perhaps there are real differences in efficacy between drugs.

Double blind, placebo (i.e., a pill without any active drug, where the patient does not know if the pill contains the drug or not) controlled drug studies are scientific studies designed to test the efficacy of pharmaceutical drugs. In these studies, the doctor administering the drug treatment doesn't know if a given patient is receiving the active drug or a placebo, and neither does the patient, thereby eliminating psychological biases in both parties. Most such drug studies of mental illness report the fraction of people who get better versus everyone else, but what about the fraction who get *worse* when given a certain drug? This is not to be confused with those who would get worse without any drug or with a placebo. The current theory predicts that Big Three drugs should in some cases make people worse, and it would be informative to understand in which instances this occurs.

A ser or nore strength adjustment with drugs may prevent relapse to overt mental illness by keeping ser or nore reset, thereby correcting brain circuitry dysfunction while simultaneously affecting Big Three traits, such as those listed in Chapter 7—so there may be these two effects.

Now let's return to the subject of The Adjustment, which is how I believe Big Three drugs should be used to improve quality of life. There already exist the six categories of FDA approved drugs to strengthen or weaken each of the Big Three, and thereby perform The Adjustment; we'll now discuss these drugs in greater detail.

Ser Strengtheners

The standard ser strengthening drugs are the SRIs (ser reuptake inhibitors): Prozac, Zoloft, Paxil, Lexapro, and Luvox. Each of these drugs is FDA approved in the United States. These are ser level boosting drugs, and they have been used successfully to treat a wide variety of overt mental illnesses, as noted by Michael Norden in *Beyond Prozac*. Though the SRIs cause general brain—and maybe throughout the rest of the body as well—boosting of ser, the ser sub-type 2A (5HT_2A) receptor may be the principal receptor that affects mental health, as My Case Study use of Zyprexa would suggest. Perhaps in the future, 5HT_2A receptor specific activators will replace the SRIs if they produce fewer side effects, such as agitation. Some people report that SRIs deaden their emotions, that they become more indifferent and less passionate while taking them. Perhaps in such cases, ser strengthening is not the appropriate adjustment.

Ser Weakeners

Ser weakening is most well established for the atypical antipsychotic drugs (which deactivate the ser 5HT_2A receptor and also deactivate dop receptors), tianeptine (a ser reuptake *enhancer* available in Europe), and cyproheptadine. The typical antipsychotic drugs, which may also weaken ser, are not as widely used now because they can cause tardive dyskinesia, a potentially irreversible movement disorder. Ser weakening is less well established for four other drugs—nefazodone, trazodone, mianserin, and ketanserin—which all deactivate the 5HT_2A receptor, but also weakly inhibit ser and/or nore reuptake, which could boost their levels and result in net ser and/or nore *strengthening*.

FDA approved atypical antipsychotics include: Clozaril, Zyprexa, Geodon, Risperdal, Seroquel, and Abilify, though the latter drug may not weaken ser. Clozaril, which is also known as clozapine, can cause a dangerous blood disorder and is not widely used. All of these drugs can cause weight gain, which may possibly be associated with Type 2 diabetes, and Geodon can affect the heart. Therefore, these are not perceived as rather benign 'recreational drugs' like the SRIs, since their side effects are more often severe. That said, these have been miracle drugs for many people with bipolar disorder and schizophrenia, and Zyprexa (along with desipramine) saved my life. These drugs may also function as antidepressants, and so they should according to The Adjustment.

Tianeptine, which is currently available in Europe and not in the United States, is a ser reuptake enhancer—thereby a weakener of ser, through reduction of its synaptic level—that has been used as an antidepressant. It could be the first drug in a new class of antidepressants that may be better tolerated than SRIs. According to my theory, tianeptine should enhance the senses and emotions in some people (particularly those who have strong ser), and these may be perceived as pleasant effects. Tianeptine may treat depression by resetting ser pathways, creating an upstream ser level change that the rest of the postsynaptic circuitry adjusts to, 'thinking' it's a new genetic level. In other words, as mentioned in Chapter 4, changing the Big Three strengths—either strengthening or weakening them—may serve to reset dysfunctional pathways to a new, healthy state. So it's not just strengthening of the Big Three that can treat depression, and this is consistent with The Adjustment. If two-thirds of depressives respond to tianeptine and two-thirds of depressives respond to a given SRI, then this implies that at least some people will respond similarly to both types of drugs, consistent with the resetting hypothesis.

Cyproheptadine, a ser 5HT_2A receptor deactivator, is another potential ser weakening drug. It is FDA approved in the United States as an antihistamine, as it also deactivates histamine receptors. Preliminary evidence suggests that it may be useful in treating depression and schizophrenia.

Nore Strengtheners

The standard nore strengthening drugs are the tricyclic antidepressant NRIs (nore reuptake inhibitors): desipramine, nortriptyline, and protriptyline. Other tricyclic antidepressants may also be NRIs, but this is unclear due to their potential additional ser boosting. A newer NRI is Strattera, which is FDA approved for treating ADHD. Another NRI, reboxetine, is available in Europe and may eventually be available in the United States. Common side effects of the tricyclics include sedation and effects on the heart, though the effects on the heart are typically not dangerous, especially in adults. Recall from My Case Study that desipramine's lone but significant side effect for me is heart arrhythmia. Because of these side effects, the nore strengthening drugs are not as popular as the SRIs for treating depression, though I believe they are underused and critical for implementing The Adjustment in some people. Maybe in the future, nore postsynaptic receptor subtype specific activators will replace the NRIs if the former drugs produce fewer side effects than the latter.

Nore Weakeners

The drugs that I propose to be nore weakeners—the alpha 2 adrenergic agonists, the alpha blockers, and the beta blockers—have not been used widely, if at all, to treat mental illness. All three types of drugs are FDA approved for heart related effects, such as lowering blood pressure and stabilizing heart rate. The alpha 2 agonists may be the most important nore weakening drugs currently available for The

Adjustment because they lower the brain level of extracellular nore—this has been shown in the rodent brain for one of these drugs, clonidine—whereas the alpha and beta blockers, if they enter the brain, may have more specific, limited effects on weakening nore that may or may not be useful for treating mental illness. In a number of preliminary studies, clonidine has been used successfully to terminate bipolar mania, though this drug has not come into widespread use for treating bipolar disorder. There's evidence that alpha 2 agonists lower the brain level of extracellular nore by binding to presynaptic nore autoreceptors in the brainstem. However, alpha 2 receptors may be present postsynaptically as well as presynaptically and if so, the alpha 2 agonists may, in some cases, strengthen nore instead of weaken it. Another possible shortcoming of these drugs is that they may only weaken nore temporarily, instead of weakening it in the long term. On the other hand, these drugs have been used to successfully treat opioid withdrawal in heroin addicts, consistent with brain nore weakening that lasts at least a few weeks, and I believe they indeed weaken nore on a long-term basis.

FDA approved alpha 2 adrenergic agonists include: clonidine, guanfacine, guanabenz acetate, and tizanidine; approved in the United Kingdom and pending United States FDA approval is lofexidine. There is a wide array of FDA approved alpha and beta blockers, including the beta blocker propranolol. In the future, perhaps nore reuptake enhancers, analogous to the ser reuptake enhancer tianeptine, can be synthesized, which will weaken nore. Furthermore, analogous to Zyprexa deactivating the ser 5HT_2A receptor and thereby weakening ser, perhaps nore weakening drugs may only need to deactivate a particular subtype of postsynaptic nore receptors—as may already be the case with certain alpha and beta blockers—to achieve their psychiatric nore weakening effect.

Finally, recall that a study of the nore weakening beta blocker propranolol indicates that nore plays a role in recognizing facial expressions of sadness. This indicates that beta blockers—and perhaps ser weakening atypical antipsychotics, tianeptine, and cyproheptadine—can exert immediate effects on the brain that could be studied in psychological experiments. Propranolol has also been used to treat migraine headaches (and so have the alpha 2 adrenergic agonists), which is consistent with beta blockers crossing the blood-brain barrier and binding to nore receptors in the brain. Preliminary evidence also indicates that propranolol can terminate bipolar mania.

Dop Strengtheners

The standard dop strengthener is the FDA approved ADHD drug, Ritalin. Two other drugs—amphetamine and cocaine—the latter of which I don't recommend using, also strengthen dop. I think the antidepressant Wellbutrin (aka Zyban) is a dop specific strengthener, though it may also strengthen nore. If Wellbutrin does strengthen nore, it would probably trigger mania in bipolar persons like ser or nore strengthening antidepressants do, but it generally does not trigger mania. And like all dop strengtheners, Wellbutrin's effects should kick in immediately—due to lack of dop saturation, and unlike the two week delay of ser and nore strengtheners—making it a unique antidepressant. However, I don't believe Wellbutrin can treat severe depression, which probably involves ser and/or nore dysfunction, but rather can provide relief to the depressed until a proper ser and/or nore drug is found, or the depression ends spontaneously. In addition, recall that The Triangle (see Chapter 5) indicates that drugs that strengthen or weaken ser and/or nore affect dop likewise.

Dop Weakeners

The standard dop weakening drugs are the atypical and typical antipsychotics (see **Ser Weakeners**), where both types of drugs may directly weaken both ser and dop by deactivating some of their receptors. Evidence that these drugs weaken dop comes not only from pharmacological animal studies but also from their efficacy in terminating bipolar mania, both in the short term and long term. Recall from My Case Study that Zyprexa, an atypical antipsychotic, terminates or at least diminishes hypomania in me. Atypical antipsychotics are now commonly used in the long-term treatment of bipolar disorder, though typical antipsychotics, such as Haldol and Thorazine, tend to only be used to terminate bipolar mania in the short term since long-term use of these drugs can cause the movement disorder tardive dyskinesia. Since there may not be a dop safety factor in place within our brain chemistry, the effect of dop weakening from antipsychotics should take place immediately.

Mixed Drugs
Tricyclic Antidepressants

The tricyclic antidepressants are a large class of drugs that have been around for over 40 years. Some of the tricyclics, in their native form, strengthen ser as well as nore through level boosting reuptake inhibition, though in the body they may only strengthen nore due to rapid breakdown into exclusively nore strengthening molecules. For example, the tricyclics amitriptyline and imipramine are rapidly metabolized in the body into nortriptyline and desipramine, respectively, which are actually NRIs. Whether all tricyclics really are nore specific is a critical question for psychopharmacology since they are a vast and potent array of drugs. If some of the tricyclics are more ser specific even when metabolized in the body, then they represent an important alternative to SRIs, maybe with more favorable side effects.

One clue as to the mechanism of a particular psychiatric drug is whether it deadens or enhances the senses, since changing the ratio of ser to nore affects sensory perception, as described in Chapter 7. For example, this would give information regarding whether all the tricyclics strengthen nore, or at least do this more so than strengthen ser. This could be tested in psychological experiments by examining how sharp or dull one's sensory perception becomes after taking these drugs, and a similar test could be applied to any putative Big Three drug, such as Wellbutrin or the monoamine oxidase inhibitors (MAOIs), where the latter drugs are a class of antidepressants that may strengthen both ser and nore.

It should also be noted that a drug that is designed to strengthen both ser and nore—such as the relatively new antidepressants Cymbalta and Effexor, and possibly some of the tricyclics—may actually only strengthen *one* in a particular person: 1) due to drug/receptor binding variability among different people, and 2) if ser and nore weaken each other strongly, as in The Triangle (see Chapter 5), then the transmitter that was boosted more strongly in a particular person would weaken the other transmitter.

Atypical Antipsychotics and Schizophrenia

Schizophrenia may actually be caused by weak or dysfunctional ser, rather than the widely believed strong dop hypothesis (discussed more in the next chapter). The atypical antipsychotics currently used to treat schizophrenia weaken both ser and dop directly. However, the direct weakening of dop may inadvertently strengthen ser according to The Triangle, and these direct and indirect effects on ser may compete with one another in a given person, and the winning effect may differ from person to person. Therefore, if schizophrenia is caused by weak ser, then the atypical antipsychotics may either improve it by strengthening ser, or make it worse by weakening ser further. If schizophrenia, however, is caused by dysfunctional ser, *any* ser strength change—either weakening or strengthening—would reset ser and thereby treat it. This may also produce the known antidepressant effect of the atypical antipsychotics. In other words, if the atypical antipsychotics make schizophrenia worse in some people, then schizophrenia may be caused by weak ser instead of dysfunctional ser. On the other hand, if ser resetting treats schizophrenia, then the SRIs can treat this illness, and so can tianeptine and cyproheptadine, which would be a landmark discovery.

Intracellular Drugs

An intracellular drug has to enter neurons as well as enter the brain to produce its therapeutic effect. The side effects of such a drug may be more favorable, and the effects more specific, than those of an external receptor binding drug. The standard treatments for bipolar disorder, namely lithium and the anticonvulsants (such as Depakote and Tegretol), appear to be intracellular drugs in that they may enter neurons and have effects on intracellular signaling cascades, rather than binding to external Big Three receptors. Because of the success of these drugs in terminating mania—where I think mania is predominantly caused by strong nore—I initially thought that they deactivate external nore receptors, but if this were the case, pharmacologists would have easily figured this out. Moreover, if lithium deactivates external nore receptors in the brain, it should have immediate psychological effects (other than sedation) like propranolol (a nore weakening beta blocker) does, but as far as I know this has never been demonstrated.

Even if lithium acts on intracellular signaling pathways, there's some evidence that its therapeutic effect may still be weakening of nore. (Of course, a drug that is intracellular may still act upon Big Three circuit strengths.) Indeed, like antidepressants, the effects of lithium and the anticonvulsants take at least a week to kick in, consistent with these drugs having an effect on ser/nore circuits. If they weaken nore, they should terminate NRI induced mania but probably not SRI induced mania, and likewise affect Big Three traits (see Chapter 7). It is also known that lithium can affect cognition, and possibly the anticonvulsants do so as well. This may be caused, via

The Triangle, by indirectly weakening dop by directly weakening nore with these drugs, since dop affects the rate and subject matter of thought, as described in Chapter 7.

LSD

The mechanism of the hallucinogenic street drug LSD has implications not only for our understanding of schizophrenia and other psychotic brain states, but also for the current theory of ser saturation that was mentioned in Chapter 4. LSD is widely considered to be an activator of postsynaptic ser receptors, probably the 5HT_2A receptor, and thereby may strengthen ser and for that reason cause psychosis. However, LSD may be a weaker activator than ser itself for the 5HT_2A receptor, thereby competing with saturated ser for binding to the receptor and thereby weakening ser transmission and causing psychosis. If LSD really does activate postsynaptic ser receptors in a manner that strengthens ser, then ser (and nore) may not really be saturated systems, due to the drug's immediate effects. One test of the theory of LSD either being a weak activator or a deactivator of the 5HT_2A receptor is that a newly synthesized drug that is a known potent *deactivator* of this receptor should produce similar hallucinogenic effects.

CHAPTER 10

OVERT MENTAL ILLNESSES

Major Points

• People with mental illness may simply have more extreme Big Three strengths than normal people; in addition, mental illness may exist with normal Big Three strengths but these transmitter systems have become dysfunctional.

• Clonidine and the other alpha 2 adrenergic agonist drugs may be superior to lithium, the anticonvulsants, and the atypical antipsychotics for the treatment of bipolar disorder.

• Prozac and the other ser reuptake inhibitor (SRI) drugs may be superior to both the typical and the atypical antipsychotics for the treatment of schizophrenia.

• Drug and alcohol abuse is a sign of low quality of life that may be treatable with The Adjustment.

In my opinion people with overt mental illnesses, that is, *DSM-IV-TR* diagnosable mental illnesses, are just more extreme Big Three variants than so called normal people. In particular, the greater a person's ser and nore strengths deviate from mid-range values, the closer that person is to having an overt mental illness, or if he suffers from a mental illness the more intense that illness is. Therefore, mental health treatment should focus upon performing The Adjustment, by adjusting ser and nore strengths with Big Three drugs closer to mid-range, optimal degrees. In addition, overt mental illness may exist with normal ser and nore strengths, but one or both of these transmitter systems has become dysfunctional and the circuitry needs to be reset with a Big Three drug or ECT, or instead non-optimal strengths and dysfunction may coexist in a given person.

Since overt mental illnesses blend into one another among different people, and drug treatments do so as well, isn't this consistent with an underlying Big Three mechanism for both? Drug based Big Three alterations such as The Adjustment may be *indirect* treatments of overt mental illnesses, but they generally are effective. Just because drug adjustment of the Big Three circuits can treat a given mental illness does not mean that illness was caused by an equal and opposite disturbance of the Big Three—these transmitters could just be inputs to other brain circuits, ways of perturbing circuits. That said, I do believe that disturbance of the Big Three systems really does *cause* at least most types of mental illness.

When, if ever, is irreversible damage done to the brain by mental illness? In the book *Against Depression*, Peter Kramer discusses evidence for damage to the brain caused by depression. Moreover, some cases of schizophrenia appear to be associated with brain atrophy. So what role, if any, does neuron death or birth play in mental illness?

Do many people have a ser deficiency, as Michael Norden has suggested in *Beyond Prozac*? Is it healthy to have as much ser as possible, or is too much of it unhealthy, as the current theory would suggest? A prevailing view is that many people are deficient in ser, but perhaps this is not the case, though I think many people have personality traits of weak ser (see Chapter 12). Another common view is that the more ser one has, the happier one is, though I don't believe that this is the case.

Many mental illnesses can be episodic in that they flare up from time to time—this is well established for unipolar depression, bipolar disorder, and schizophrenia. Are all mental illnesses actually episodic, or at least not constant over time?

Maybe the brain repels overt mental illnesses—induced by stress or other, possibly natural stimuli—all the time, and only in a few cases, perhaps in susceptible individuals, do we see it break through. Perhaps there are many near misses.

In reading about the specific mental illnesses below, the reader will notice that the most common Big Three strength combination in these illnesses is weak ser and/or strong nore, which is a recurring theme in this book. According to the The Adjustment theory, people with this pair of strengths would best be treated by using two drugs simultaneously: one drug that strengthens weak ser and another drug that weakens strong nore. Other people will only need one drug, because only ser is weak or nore is strong. See Chapters 8 and 9 for details on which drugs to use and how to use them in this manner, as well as for treating other combinations of pathological Big Three strengths.

Depression
Causes and Treatments

Depression may be caused by non-optimal strengths of ser and/or nore, the dysfunction of ser/nore circuits, or both of these phenomena. If dysfunction is necessary for depression, then non-optimal ser and/or nore strengths can also contribute by making the depression more intense. Indeed, strong ser and nore should be just as pathological as weak ser and nore in exacerbating depression, even though psychiatrists typically only use ser and/or nore strengthening antidepressants to treat it. Recall that the ser weakening drug tianeptine treats depression, and the antidepressant effect of the atypical antipsychotics may also be mediated by ser weakening. So resetting of ser/nore circuitry—in most cases through a level change—may be the universal feature of antidepressants and ECT. For these reasons, I think of lack of depression as a logical AND (introduced in Chapter 6) for the ser and nore systems, where both systems must be functional and at mid-range, optimal strengths to produce optimal mood.

So are there ser or nore specific depressions? Possibly. And how does OR circuit modulation relate to this? OR logic implies that any drug that optimizes (or at least strengthens or weakens) ser or nore will reset the depression circuits and treat the illness— however, this is argued against by a study that shows ser strengthening without an antidepressant effect in some depressed persons. OR also implies that a ser drug or a nore drug should both work in the same person, and is argued for by the fact that SRIs and NRIs each work in about 70% of depressed people—with these percentages many people should respond well to either class of drugs. This sort of reasoning in favor of OR leads to the conclusion that practically any ser and/or nore drug can treat depression, including the typical antipsychotics (if they all indeed weaken ser), the alpha 2 adrenergic agonists such as clonidine, and the 5HT_2A receptor deactivators such as cyproheptadine. So while I acknowledge that treating depression as a logical OR for ser and nore drug manipulations is promising and deserves more scientific attention, I still think that ser AND nore must be at mid-range, non-dysfunctional strengths for optimal mood, and this must be considered during drug treatment.

Though we may use a simple ser AND nore drug treatment strategy for attacking all depressions, there may still be different types of depressions, with different underlying Big Three neurotransmitter system abnormalities, that require different drug regimens in order to render ser AND nore at optimal, mid-range strengths. If so, maybe these depressions can be distinguished in terms of their effects on sleep, appetite, and diurnal (within the day) fluctuation in mood. One well known subtype of depression is atypical depression, which is characterized by: oversleeping and overeating, mood brightening transiently in response to positive external events, sensitivity to interpersonal rejection, and heavy, leaden feelings in the arms and legs. Perhaps in the majority of cases atypical depression involves weak ser (and strong nore), since it has been shown to respond better to SRIs than to NRIs. However, if strong nore is part of the pathology, NRIs should actually make the depression *worse*, and nore weakening drugs such as clonidine should treat it. A further test of atypical depression involving strong nore is whether such people have personality traits of strong nore.

Two other potential subtypes of depression that are very likely an oversimplification: undersleeping signifies severe depression, and oversleeping signifies mild or moderate depression. My Case Study is an example that the same person can oversleep and undersleep at different times during the course of treatment for depression, though I underslept during my most severe depression and overslept during milder depression.

Another potential subtype of depression is psychotic depression, during which the individual experiences hallucinations and/or delusions, as well as a depressed mood. Psychotic depression may respond better to SRIs than to NRIs, similar to atypical depression, since psychosis may be caused by weak or dysfunctional ser, or a low ser/nore strength ratio, consistent with my proposed mechanism of the hallucinogen, LSD (see Chapter 9), which itself causes psychosis. Moreover, if psychosis is caused by a low ser/nore ratio, then NRIs should make psychotic depression worse.

Most people with depression feel better as the day wears on, though some feel worse, and these are two other potential subtypes of depression. Keep in mind that since, as described in Chapter 4, ser and nore build as the day wears on, depressions that get better or worse as the day wears on may have something to do with this putative transmitter build-up. I think depressions that get worse as the day wears on are due to build-up of nore, and should respond to nore weakening and/or ser strengthening drugs and not the opposite adjustments.

Whether a particular person's depression lowers self-esteem may be a clue to the underlying Big Three abnormality, since ser (and dop) strength partially encode self-esteem (see Chapter 7).

Can everyone become depressed with a great enough stressor? Possibly, though perhaps expanded dysthymics (discussed in the next chapter), who suffer from constant mild depression, are more likely to be affected. The continuum theory for depression, namely that the less optimal a person's strengths of ser and nore, the greater the severity of her depression, is consistent with the hypothesis that some people are 'farther away from depression' than others if their Big Three systems are better optimized. And maybe depression is more common in dysthymics if mild depression is more likely to set off a snowballing effect involving escalating responses to stressors that eventually results in more severe depression.

Relationship to Stress

Stress is thought to be a cause of depression—and other types of mental illness—in at least some cases. A possible mechanism is that stress causes a massive release of the Big Three from their brainstem neurons, followed by a diminished release of these transmitters, leading to subsequent dysfunction and/or abnormally low strengths of the Big Three, especially ser and/or nore. However, summary data from the book by Frederick Goodwin and Kay Redfield Jamison, *Manic-Depressive Illness*, suggest that lower levels of the Big Three during depression may only be the case for dop. But, if depression is *totally* caused by weak dop, then cocaine, Ritalin, and amphetamine should totally reverse it, at least temporarily, but they do not.

Speaking of stress, which aspects of American society contribute to causing depression by increasing stress on the individual? Theory: 1) non-nomadic living conditions, 2) isolated living conditions, 3) isolated working conditions, 4) unnaturally stressful work itself, and 5) availability of too much information.

Two Week Delay

Finally, the two week delay in response to antidepressants—and many other Big Three drugs—is one of the principal reasons researchers have strayed from the Big Three/biogenic amine *level* hypothesis of depression, but this delay can easily be explained by the internal regulation of the postsynaptic circuitry, where a safety factor in the pathway renders the circuit unresponsive to an immediate boosting of ser and/or nore (see Chapter 4 for more details).

Bipolar Disorder
Typical and Atypical

Psychiatry already recognizes at least two subtypes of bipolar disorder: bipolar I and bipolar II, which involve episodes of full-blown mania (bipolar I) and mild mania (hypomania; bipolar II), interspersed with episodes of depression. So bipolar I is the more severe of the two subtypes. I think there are at least two other subtypes of bipolar disorder—typical and atypical—that may each contain individuals with bipolar I and bipolar II. I refer to typical bipolar disorder as 'typical' because it is by far the most common of the two subtypes—perhaps 100 times more common than atypical bipolar disorder, based on the personality characteristics of bipolar persons I have known or known about. Typical bipolar disorder is characterized by genetically strong nore and weak ser, whereas atypical bipolar disorder is characterized by genetically strong ser and weak nore. The existence of typical and atypical bipolar disorder follows directly from The Triangle (see Chapter 5), since genetically strong ser or strong nore tends to produce the strong dop that is characteristic of mania/hypomania.

In addition to the standard manic symptoms listed in the *DSM-IV-*

TR, typical (strong nore, strong dop) mania may be distinguished from atypical (strong ser, strong dop) mania in that typical mania may produce: decreased need for sleep, presence of hallucinations and/or delusions, heightening of the five senses, and decreased sensitivity to the cold. In contrast, atypical mania (as in My Case Study) may produce: decreased sleep (without feeling rested), absence of hallucinations and delusions, deadening of the five senses, and increased sensitivity to the cold. Both types of mania may result in reduced emotional sensitivity, and strengthened dop may be the cause of this insensitivity. If ser and dop encode self-esteem, then the atypical bipolars/hypomanics may have the highest self-esteem of anyone, though typical bipolars/hypomanics may also have high self-esteem due to strong dop.

So the cause of typical mania/hypomania is that the strength of nore has increased—possibly due to an environmental trigger such as stress, and always accompanied by strong genetic nore—causing the dop strength to also increase (as in The Triangle), and it is this elevated dop strength that causes most of the symptoms. (Recall that cocaine, a dop strengthener, produces a high that is similar to that in mania.) As the nore and dop strengths increase, they weaken ser (also described in The Triangle), and it is this weakened ser (or low ser/nore ratio) that causes the hallucinations and delusions present in typical mania.

Atypical mania/hypomania (as in My Case Study) is similar except it involves strong ser instead of strong nore. It is possible that atypical mania can only be induced in people by ser strengthening drugs such as the SRIs, since very strong genetic ser is so rare, whereas typical mania can have either external (such as drugs or seasons) or internal (such as genetics) causes. Atypical antipsychotics, which directly weaken ser and dop, are ideal for treating atypical mania, though they can also treat the strong dop aspect of typical mania.

Both subtypes of bipolar disorder seem to involve pathological imbalances of ser and nore, in which one is strong and the other is weak, based on the personality characteristics of bipolar persons I have known or known about. And the greater the imbalance of ser and nore, the greater the pathology, which follows from The Adjustment theory itself. Therefore, if nearly all or all bipolar people (and many people who are hypomanic all the time) have a pathological ser/nore imbalance, then use of a drug such as an antidepressant that strengthens the weak one as well as a drug that weakens the strong one should be standard treatment (as in My Case Study), though adding antidepressants in bipolar treatment remains controversial because many of these drugs can trigger mania or rapid mood cycling.

Furthermore, due to this putative ser/nore imbalance that may exist whether the person's mood is cycling or is not (due to a mood stabilizing drug), perhaps a lot of bipolar persons are non-compliant with their medication, in that they stop taking their medication without approval from their doctor, not only because they miss being hypomanic—if they indeed have stopped cycling—but also because their quality of life is lower than a 'normal' person's quality of life. Such poorer quality of life—a type of expanded dysthymia, discussed in the next chapter—may be the case even though psychiatrists may tell the person that life on medication is what it's like to be normal, when in fact they are not on the proper regimen of medication at all: a proper regimen would involve performing The Adjustment. So maybe for bipolar II disorder (in which the person is continuously cycling), mild cycling may be a better treatment option than total stoppage of cycling—if total stoppage is even possible—since the person may crave hypomania and be non-compliant without it.

As stated in Chapter 9, perhaps clonidine and the other alpha 2 adrenergic agonists only weaken nore in the short term and not in the long term due to drug adaptation by the brain. But if these drugs do indeed weaken nore in the long term—and I think they do—they could be landmark drugs for (typical) bipolar disorder (especially when used in conjunction with a ser strengthening drug). Indeed, the alpha 2 agonists may be superior mood stabilizers, in their overall effect on quality of life, than lithium, the anticonvulsants, the atypical antipsychotics, and the typical antipsychotics, particularly if lithium and the anticonvulsants don't weaken nore.

Bipolar I and Bipolar II

Bipolar I and bipolar II are the two well-established subtypes of bipolar disorder, where bipolar I is characterized by full-blown episodes of mania and bipolar II has episodes of hypomania. These two subtypes may in fact be related to one another as a continuum among different people, just as mania to hypomania or atypical to typical bipolar disorder may be continua, though if bipolar I and bipolar II have different seasonal patterns—which they probably don't in all cases—they may really represent two categories.

Do people with bipolar I or bipolar II disorder ever really stop mood cycling? The conventional wisdom is that people with bipolar I have normal moods between manias and depressions and people with bipolar II don't.

It would be consistent with the so-called permissive hypothesis of mania, which states that weak genetic ser 'permits' induction of full-blown mania in people with bipolar disorder, if bipolar II people tend to have stronger ser than bipolar I people, since those with bipolar I have full-blown episodes of mania. However, the permissive hypothesis probably isn't true, just based on the personality traits of bipolars I've known who had very weak ser without full-blown mania, making them bipolar II and not bipolar I. Moreover, the permissive hypothesis is argued against by the general finding that SRIs induce mania in bipolars. A variant of the permissive hypothesis that may be true: genetically weak ser is necessary but not sufficient for full-blown mania.

One clear principle in the drug treatment of all subtypes of bipolar disorder is that they should either be treated with a mood stabilizer, or a mood stabilizer and an antidepressant, but never with an antidepressant alone, since an antidepressant alone will induce mania and/or rapid, pathological mood cycling. So does increasing the dose of standard mood stabilizer, such as lithium and the anticonvulsants, turn bipolar I into bipolar II in a given person? And does increasing the dose of an antidepressant do the opposite? In both cases: probably not, as if there are hardwired, largely genetic brain differences between the two bipolar subtypes. For treating bipolar depression, especially bipolar II depression, one may never need to use a higher dose of an antidepressant (in conjunction with a mood stabilizer, of course) than that which makes one hypomanic. Higher doses may produce pathological, rapid mood cycling (as in My Case Study).

Brain Mechanisms

Big Three drugs—and lithium and the anticonvulsants, possibly— affect the frequency (how often it occurs) and amplitude (how severe it is) of bipolar disorder mood cycling, as well as other perceptual phenomena, such as how sharp one's five senses are, associated with depression and mania. In My Case Study, strengthening weak nore and weakening strong ser (i.e., The Adjustment) made my hypomanias more enjoyable and my depressions less pathological.

For people with bipolar disorder, an episode of mania or hypomania is usually followed by a crash into depression, and then the cycle repeats. So bipolar disorder may involve a 'switch in the brain' for shutting off mania/hypomania and turning on depression, a function which every brain has but in most individuals is never invoked because they never get—or are incapable of getting—manic or hypomanic. The switch may have different thresholds in different people, explaining the existence of constant hypomanics. In other words, people who are constantly hypomanic may have a high threshold for their switch, such that they remain hypomanic all the time. Likewise, there may be a switch for shutting off depression and turning on mania/hypomania.

In My Case Study, the transition from hypomania to depression was sometimes instantaneous, though for most people gradual transitions are probably the norm. Nonetheless, what does *instantaneous* switching tell one about Big Three strengths changing as the putative switching mechanism? This may rule out Big Three brain extracellular level changing—which should be relatively slow—as the mechanism. Similarly, do the Big Three 'push a swinging gate' in the brain circuitry, that flips from on (mania) to off (depression) with potentially rapid, or even instantaneous, transitions between the two states, or is there no such gate in bipolar disorder? What does immediate termination of mania by dop weakeners tell one about this? And if bipolar disorder involves multiple brain circuits—in other words, multiple parallel processes—these circuits may have different rates at which they cycle, such that they are not synchronous. For example, at a given time, the circuits that control sensory sharpness may be affected differently than the circuits that control the subject matter of thought.

If mania involves strong ser or nore—as well as strong dop—can it really be terminated immediately by just a dop weakener? Apparently it can be. Moreover, is the mechanism of terminating mania different for lithium, the anticonvulsants, and the anti-psychotics? If it is, this is a clue regarding the mechanisms underlying mania and the mechanisms of these drugs.

Ultra-rapid cycling bipolar disorder, in which mood—or at least emotion—fluctuates dramatically within a single day, may be caused by super strong nore, or a high nore/ser ratio, possibly interacting with particular hardwired circuits. In other words, if strong nore plays an important role in producing emotions (see Chapter 7), weakening nore may result in a type of mood stabilization, independent of and confused with stabilizing standard bipolar disorder.

Perhaps the default for some bipolar people is to *always* get manic when taking no drugs—though this may be subsequently followed by depression—whereas the default for others is to *always* get depressed when taking no drugs, as in My Case Study. Perhaps this is an important distinction that requires different approaches to drug treatment. In other words, the always manic type may not require an antidepressant but only a mood stabilizer, whereas the always depressed type may require both an antidepressant and a mood stabilizer.

In mood cycling we must distinguish between internal causes (produced by a combination of genetics and past experience) and external causes (such as the seasons, drugs, stress, possibly other recent environmental conditions such as sleep deprivation). Along these lines, to what extent can the individual affect the cycling of his own mood? In particular, can the individual push himself for a number of days and then cause a subsequent depression? It should be noted that sleep deprivation can induce mania, and a person can, to some extent, also regulate exposure to stress.

What does it mean that even tiny doses of antidepressants induce mania/hypomania in bipolar individuals, even, as in My Case Study, for a stress induced depression? It is as if the antidepressant is working on a stage in the cortical circuitry that is different from the one that the stress altered, or is just resetting the circuitry.

Additional Observations

Why is bipolar disorder a predictor of wealth? (Note: for a discussion of this subject, see Goodwin and Jamison's *Manic-Depressive Illness*.) For example, since most bipolar persons have both periods of depression and periods of mania, and if these ups and downs balance each other out, a bipolar person should be average—in terms of productivity, income, etc.—yet often they are not. This implies that even while depressed (or in a mixed mood), many bipolar people have above average energy (and/or possibly above average intellect). On the other hand, many bipolar individuals are occupationally impaired due to their disorder.

What does the genetic relatedness of bipolar disorder and unipolar depression (i.e., a mental illness in which people only have depression) mean with respect to the Big Three (aka, biogenic amine or chemical imbalance) theory of depression and mania, particularly with regard to the genetic strengths of the Big Three? Indeed, the offspring/relatives of unipolar depressives not only have elevated rates of unipolar depression but also have elevated rates of bipolar disorder, and the offspring/relatives of bipolars not only have elevated rates of bipolar disorder but also elevated rates of unipolar depression. The biogenic amine theory would predict that the two illnesses be *anticorrelated* among different relatives, since low levels of the Big Three should produce depression and high levels should produce mania. In other words, the biogenic amine theory would predict that the offspring/relatives of unipolar depressives have very low rates of bipolar disorder (and vice versa), due to the inheritance of genes encoding low levels of the Big Three. However, this may not be the case if there is often an underlying imbalance of ser and nore—one strong and the other weak—in both bipolar disorder and unipolar depression. If typical bipolar disorder involves strong nore and so does atypical depression, do depressed relatives of typical bipolars show atypical depressive features? Finally, if bipolar disorder really has a nearly 100% concordance rate between identical twins, which means that when one twin has the disorder, the other twin nearly always does as well, as has been reported, then perhaps it isn't usually brought on by unusual stress, though it may be exacerbated by stress.

Seasonal Affective Disorder (SAD)

SAD is a common disorder that is characterized by seasonal changes in mood, in most cases by wintertime depression. The relationship between SAD and bipolar disorder is unclear, as bipolar disorder also in many cases has a seasonal pattern, often with wintertime depression. There may be partial overlap in the occurrence of SAD and bipolar disorder among different people, and if so this would be another example of mental illnesses blending together. It would be interesting if *all* bipolar disorders turn out to be seasonal—or at least have a seasonal component or shift in the average degree of depression or mania. Alternatively, SAD may be a special type of bipolar disorder. And perhaps other mental illnesses, particularly unipolar depression, have a seasonal component.

If the cause of wintertime depression in SAD is mediated by seasonal changes in light, is it mediated by: the total amount of light exposure over many days, just the peak intensity of light delivered for a very short amount of time each day, the rate of change of the length of day as the seasons change, or the absolute length of daylight in different seasons? All are obvious points that researchers of SAD have probably considered. However, My Case Study indicates that bright light therapy, which is the standard treatment of SAD, does not necessarily reverse wintertime depression, but instead simply strengthens ser. Therefore, the cause of wintertime depression may not involve light at all, but rather some other external (such as temperature) or internal (such as a biological clock, analogous to a circadian rhythm) signal. Moreover, bright light therapy may strengthen ser in everyone, not just those with SAD, and may be effective in all seasons—which would be a landmark discovery for the treatment of mental illness, especially depression. In other words, bright light therapy may not be producing an effect that is equal and opposite to the cause of seasonal depression—it may have an antidepressant effect with a different, independent mechanism of action, such as ser strengthening. One study indicates that personality changes associated with bright light therapy are consistent with ser strengthening.

According to another study, bright light therapy for SAD does not boost Big Three transmitter *levels*, indicative of an antidepressant effect independent of level boosting, which might represent a separate brain mechanism that could be capitalized upon by new types of antidepressant drugs. But even if the ser level isn't boosted, the ser circuitry could still be strengthened. And evidence from My Case Study is consistent with ser level boosting: bright light therapy upset my gut, made my hands cold and shaky, and produced a state of hypomania similar to that induced by Zoloft.

Another possible treatment for SAD is dawn simulation via a light in the bedroom that gradually gets brighter as dawn approaches. One study indicates that dawn simulation is superior to bright light therapy in treating wintertime depression. As in bright light therapy for SAD, the variables of dawn simulation may be critical: time of morning, duration of light exposure each day, light spectrum, and light intensity.

If SAD was selected for by evolution to regulate seasonal behavior, and may be critical to the survival and reproduction of the individual, then maybe it is produced by a combination of several brain mechanisms, since a single brain mechanism may be less reliable. These mechanisms could include more than one of: an internal clock, temperature change, light change, or any other physiologically detectible seasonal difference. The less common, and the less essential for survival and reproduction the SAD, the less likely that it is mediated by several mechanisms, and the more likely it would be responsive to a single type of treatment such as bright light therapy.

Here's a possible experiment that would provide clues to the brain mechanism of SAD: what happens when someone with wintertime depression moves from the northern hemisphere to the southern hemisphere, or vice versa, since the timing of the seasons reverses? Does his depression shift to the new wintertime? If SAD is based on an internal clock then there may be no shift of seasons, but if SAD really is based on external wintertime cues then it should shift.

If the SAD mechanism turns out to be a ser or nore level change (and maybe even if it is instead a strength change elsewhere in the ser/nore brain circuitry), it can probably be compensated for by increasing the dose of antidepressant during the wintertime—or in the summertime, in the case of SAD with summertime depression. However, flux due to changes in types of drugs and/or their dosages (see Chapter 9) may make seasonal changes in their use decrease rather than increase quality of life.

Finally, people diagnosed with SAD, who are responsive to bright light therapy, may actually represent at least two categories of patients: those who are very sensitive to ambient lighting throughout the year and have a lower mood during the wintertime since there is less sunlight, and those who are not sensitive to ambient lighting (as in My Case Study) but nonetheless have a decrease in average mood during the wintertime. The first category of patients may be immediate responders to bright light therapy, whereas patients in the second category may take a week or more of bright light therapy before experiencing an improvement in mood (a timecourse that is similar to taking an antidepressant drug).

Schizophrenia
Causes and Treatments

Since the advent of antipsychotic drug treatment in the 1950s, it has been widely hypothesized that schizophrenia is caused by strong dop, since dop weakening antipsychotic drugs terminate its psychosis. However, a recent study has shown that typical antipsychotics, such as Haldol and Thorazine, directly weaken ser as well as dop, as do the atypical antipsychotics, such as Zyprexa and Geodon, so the actual neural basis of schizophrenia may be based in ser rather than dop. And even though therapeutic response (how much better the patient gets) to typical antipsychotics correlates with how well these drugs bind to the dop D2 receptor, maybe therapeutic response also correlates with how well they bind to the ser 5HT_2A receptor, which I think is the principal ser receptor involved in mental illness. In addition, according to The Triangle (see Chapter 5), dop weakens ser, so perhaps when antipsychotics weaken dop this strengthens ser, thereby strengthening weak ser and/or resetting dysfunctional ser circuitry.

Here are some more arguments against schizophrenia being caused by strong dop (where traits 2–5 would be mediated by strong dop): 1) dop neurons do not send connections as strongly to sensory cortex (which should be involved in hallucinations) as they do to prefrontal cortex; 2) schizophrenics don't have dominant traits, and bipolars do—measured in wealth alone, though there are many exceptions; 3) they don't have racing thoughts—in fact, they tend to have poverty (i.e., diminishment) of thought or derailment (i.e., wandering) of thought, consistent with hypofrontality; 4) they don't have stimulus seeking traits; 5) they don't have high energy or exhibit hyperactivity; and 6) antipsychotic drugs terminate psychosis after weeks, not minutes, even though dop weakening occurs in minutes and there is no dop safety factor.

The current theory hypothesizes that schizophrenia is actually caused by weak and/or dysfunctional ser rather than strong dop (or strong ser), for the reasons listed above and since: 1) the street drug LSD, which may weaken ser (see Chapter 9), produces hallucinations, delusions, paranoia, catatonia (paralysis of movement), insomnia, and derailment of thought; 2) ser is distributed throughout the thinking (prefrontal) and sensory regions of the brain, whereas dop is more concentrated just in the thinking region of the brain. If schizophrenia is indeed caused by weak ser, then SRIs such as Prozac should treat both its positive symptoms (such as hallucinations, delusions, and disorganized speech) and its negative symptoms (such as lingering apathy, emotional flattening, and poverty of speech), and this would be a landmark discovery and improvement in treatment. Moreover, the negative symptoms are consistent with expanded dysthymia (discussed in the next chapter) due to weak ser. Derailment of thought and disorganized thought or speech may be due to lack of a ser filter for filtering out irrelevant details. Consistent with weak or dysfunctional ser causing schizophrenia, a genetics study has revealed a chromosomal region associated with susceptibility "not only for schizophrenia but also for anxiety-related personality traits such as harm avoidance and neuroticism". Moreover, alleles (variants of a gene) of the 5HT_2A receptor have been directly associated with schizophrenia. Schizophrenics can also exhibit autistic symptoms, sharpened senses, and enhanced musical ability, as described in Sol Snyder's classic book, *Madness and the Brain*—all consistent with weak ser (and in the latter two of these traits, consistent with strong nore). Schizophrenia often coexists with obsessive-compulsive disorder (OCD), and OCD is often treatable with SRIs. Finally, the schizophrenics I've met have the personality characteristics of weak ser, not strong ser or strong dop, though some have strong nore characteristics as well.

LSD psychosis mimics schizophrenia far better than cocaine or amphetamine psychosis, or ketamine or PCP ('angel dust') psychosis, where these latter four drugs are often thought to produce stuporous states that resemble schizophrenia. Cocaine or amphetamine psychosis is a poor model of schizophrenia for several reasons, since these drugs: 1) produce hyperactivity rather than catatonia; 2) produce euphoria rather than apathy or depression; 3) produce racing, related thoughts rather than derailment and poverty of thought; 4) produce excessive speech rather than poverty of speech; and 5) produce a much less delusional state than schizophrenia. However, it's possible that *long-term* use of cocaine or amphetamine can induce a state of psychosis that is more similar to that in schizophrenia. In addition, NMDA receptor (which is a brain receptor for the neurotransmitter glutamate) binding drugs, such as ketamine and PCP, are also poor models of schizophrenia, although these drugs can produce a stuporous state resembling catatonia, though so can LSD.

An alternative to the strong dop and weak ser hypotheses is that schizophrenia is produced by strong nore. If so, schizophrenia, like typical bipolar disorder, should be more prevalent among artists— who I hypothesize to be strong in nore (see Chapter 12)—than among the general population. I think strong nore is the distant second best explanation for schizophrenia after weak or dysfunctional ser, mainly because of LSD, which seems to be specific to ser. Moreover, the effectiveness of dop weakening antipsychotics in treating schizophrenia may also be inconsistent with schizophrenia being caused by strong nore, since due to The Triangle weakening dop should *strengthen* nore and make the psychosis worse. Nonetheless, weak ser producing psychosis may be a special case of a low ser/nore ratio producing psychosis. If schizophrenia is indeed produced by a low ser/nore ratio, then the most effective treatment, according to The Adjustment, is to strengthen ser with an SRI drug such as Prozac, and simultaneously weaken nore with an alpha 2 adrenergic agonist drug such as clonidine.

A possible experiment: add an SRI, an NRI, or Ritalin (a dop strengthener) to the standard antipsychotic regimen of schizophrenics. How do these Big Three manipulations affect the positive or negative symptoms of the illness? Next experiment: compare an SRI to tianeptine or cyproheptadine, which are ser weakeners. Tianeptine and cyproheptadine could, like an SRI, reset dysfunctional ser circuits, though I think the SRIs should produce an overall superior effect. As mentioned above, if schizophrenia is affected by nore, alpha 2 adrenergic agonists such as clonidine should affect its outcome, and preliminary data support this hypothesis. Moreover, preliminary data indicate that the nore weakening beta blocker propranolol may have some efficacy in treating schizophrenia.

Brain structural abnormalities, such as general atrophy, that have been associated with some cases of schizophrenia may be caused by long-term Big Three abnormalities, or long-term consequences of the illness itself.

Comparison with Other Psychotic States

On a more general note, are there systematic differences in the psychosis between schizophrenia, typical mania, and psychotic depression, even if all three illnesses are at least partially caused by weak or dysfunctional ser? For example, are the characteristics of paranoia or hallucinations different in these three illnesses, as this may provide evidence as to whether they have a common cause? Perhaps a similar Big Three drug treatment, such as the SRIs or tianeptine, can be used for all three illnesses. And if schizophrenia drugs, such as the atypical antipsychotics, can treat mania, can mania drugs (lithium, anticonvulsants) treat schizophrenia?

I'm not suggesting that schizophrenia should no longer be treated with the standard antipsychotic drugs, but rather that ser resetting or strengthening may be the actual basis of such treatment, and that further research should be conducted to test this hypothesis. So it's possible that the SRIs are the best available drugs for treating schizophrenia, both for treating its positive and its negative symptoms, and this would be a landmark breakthrough for the treatment of this illness (especially considering that treatment of the illness with existing antipsychotic drugs is often not very effective). There's already ample evidence that the SRIs can treat its negative symptoms, which may be due to weak ser as well as weak dop, and there's preliminary evidence that these drugs can treat its positive symptoms as well.

Attention Deficit Hyperactivity Disorder (ADHD)

The current theory puts forth two alternative hypotheses for the cause of ADHD: 1) prefrontal hypofrontality (i.e., poor functioning of this part of the brain) due to weak dop, where according to The Triangle (see Chapter 5), weak dop may be caused by weak ser and/or weak nore; 2) sensory-emotional hypersensitivity due to weak ser and perhaps strong nore. I think 1) is the more credible hypothesis, partly because hypofrontality may explain the characteristic hyperactivity due to lack of planning of movement, since the prefrontal cortex is involved in such planning. In other words, people with ADHD may be reacting immediately to nearly every incoming stimulus in their environment or their thoughts, instead of having more calculated, selective reactions to these stimuli based on a consistent plan of action. In ADHD individuals, cocaine and amphetamines, which are dop strengtheners, cause focus, not euphoria, consistent with these people having hypofrontality. In other words, these drugs restore normal functioning to prefrontal cortex in people with ADHD, though I'm not suggesting that people with ADHD should use cocaine. A possible experiment: give ADHD individuals: 1) an SRI, 2) an NRI, 3) Ritalin (a dop strengthener), 4) both an SRI and an NRI, and see which treatment is best.

In *Shadow Syndromes*, Ratey and Johnson point out that people with ADHD can be quite successful, always seeking the next stimulus. Stimulus seeking behavior may also be related to strong dop according to Cloninger (see Chapter 12); so whether weak or strong, dop may be implicated in stimulus seeking. As we'll discuss in Chapter 13, dop can also affect dominance, so what is the relationship between ADHD, hypofrontality, and dominance? Even though I hypothesize that dop is usually strong in dominant individuals, the stimulus seeking aspects of ADHD may also produce dominant characteristics. Nonetheless, at least some aspects of cognition are impaired in ADHD, and this may diminish dominance.

ADHD can be confused with or coexist with depression—another example of mental illnesses blending into one another—and it may also be confused with bipolar disorder, since mania/hypomania due to bipolar disorder may mimic some of the symptoms of ADHD, such as inability to concentrate and hyperactivity. ADHD also blends into Tourette's syndrome, where both illnesses are characterized by impulsiveness. Obsessive-compulsive disorder (OCD) also appears to blend with both illnesses, and clonidine (a nore weakener) is a standard treatment for Tourette's.

Anxiety

Anxiety is a feeling of which we are consciously aware, and anxiety disorders probably evolved, like other mental illnesses, to drive behavior in various ways. It is not surprising that anxiety often occurs in people with weak ser (and possibly strong nore), since some weak ser people may fulfill a personality niche associated with hypervigilance, including having acute senses. In other words, such people are constantly scanning the environment for signs of danger, and this may have aided in their survival during the course of evolution. It is less clear to me why anxiety often coexists with depression, though an overlap in brain circuitry may be involved. If some people are incredibly anxious, maybe some people are pathologically calm, as in people with super strong ser and/or super weak nore.

We can classify the overt anxiety disorders as either long-standing or transient. Both genetically weak ser and strong nore may play a role in these disorders, though the role of weak ser may be more important. So the most effective treatment for them all, according to The Adjustment, is to strengthen ser with an SRI drug such as Prozac, and simultaneously weaken nore with an alpha 2 adrenergic agonist drug such as clonidine.

Long-standing anxiety disorders: agoraphobia, specific phobias, social phobia, generalized anxiety disorder, and obsessive-compulsive disorder (OCD). In most cases, the disorder has been present for nearly all of the individual's life, or at least nearly all of their adult life.

Transient anxiety disorders: panic attacks, panic disorder, post-traumatic stress disorder, and acute stress disorder. Principal cause: genetically weak ser that has been made weaker and/or dysfunctional by environmental stress, and possibly strong and/or dysfunctional nore. In most cases, the disorder has only been present since the stressful event.

Alpha 2 adrenergic antagonists (such as yohimbine and idazoxan), which probably strengthen nore, increase anxiety and arousal, whereas alpha 2 adrenergic agonists such as clonidine, which probably weaken nore, can reduce anxiety and arousal. Neither class of drugs is currently widely used for psychiatric purposes in the United States. In addition, the nore weakening beta blocker propranolol has been shown to decrease anxiety in preliminary studies.

Generalized anxiety disorder may be caused by weak ser and/or strong nore, consistent with sensory-emotional hypersensitivity (see Chapter 7). It may be paradoxical that individuals with weak ser and strong nore are in many cases anxious, because of the role of strong nore in some cases of dominance (see Chapter 13).

SRIs, NRIs, and MAOIs—the latter of which probably strengthen ser and nore—all treat panic attacks (but in the same person?). This is paradoxical if nore strengthening drugs such as the NRIs can also increase general anxiety—perhaps panic attacks and general anxiety are mediated by different Big Three circuits. Likewise, propranolol and clonidine, putative nore weakeners, also treat panic attacks. Maybe resetting of dysfunctional nore is the mechanism for all of these nore drugs in treating such attacks. So both ser and nore may be involved in panic attacks—an AND in the ser/nore circuits, in that both systems have to be intact in order to be free of the attacks.

Anxiety also appears to be quelled by dop. Cigarette smoking, which strengthens dop, tends to quell anxiety. Also the drug Zyban, which may strengthen dop and is chemically identical to Wellbutrin, is effective in helping people quit smoking.

Historically, two classes of drugs—the barbiturates and the benzodiazepines (such as Valium, Klonopin, and Xanax)—have been the standard treatments for general anxiety, and both classes of drugs bind to GABA receptors in the brain. GABA is the brain's principal inhibitory neurotransmitter, and by binding to GABA receptors these drugs quell neural activity throughout the brain in a very general manner. I believe that affecting GABA receptors is an indirect treatment of anxiety, which is caused by weak ser and/or strong nore, and should ideally be treated with ser and nore drugs. In contrast, the barbiturates and benzodiazepines provide a poorer treatment, since they are addictive, require increasingly higher doses to maintain their effect, and produce a 'drugged' feeling.

Drug and Alcohol Abuse

Psychologists have long recognized that a particular pattern of behavior, such as alcohol abuse, is likely to become a habit if that behavior produces an overall positive experience in the individual. This implies that a mentally healthy, happy person could, if the stimulus is positive enough, succumb to drug and alcohol abuse, though I think this is rarely the case—instead, drug and alcohol abuse is almost always a sign of Big Three strength abnormality and/or dysfunction. In other words, I think in almost all cases people self-medicate when their quality of life is lower than normal—in that they exhibit expanded dysthymia, described in the next chapter—and the drug or alcohol produces a significant improvement in quality of life.

Therefore, a large fraction of drug and alcohol addicts would benefit from The Adjustment. The most common Big Three profile among drug and alcohol abusers is probably weak ser and/or strong nore.

Drug and alcohol abuse is also very common in overtly mentally ill individuals, such as those with unipolar depression, bipolar disorder, or anxiety disorders. Weak dop—and strong dop, as in mania and hypomania—has been strongly associated with addictive behavior.

Personality Disorders

The personality disorders include a broad range of psychiatric illnesses in which the individual probably experiences the world in a deviant manner and also exhibits various types of deviant behavior. These disorders may in part involve hardwired circuits that aren't affected by Big Three adjustments—this is the conventional wisdom, but I don't believe it's correct. Instead, I think the personality disorders are actually caused by genetically weak ser (and/or strong nore) interacting with hardwired circuits. So I think they can be treated somewhat by Big Three drugs, and early intervention may be preferable if there really is a developmental component to these disorders.

Personality disorders caused by weak ser (and possibly strong nore): paranoid, schizoid, schizotypal, antisocial, borderline, avoidant, dependent, and obsessive-compulsive. Those caused by strong nore (and possibly weak ser): histrionic and narcissistic. These latter two disorders may be related to Cloninger's strong nore reward dependence trait, discussed in Chapter 12.

Autism

The current theory hypothesizes that autism is caused by developmentally weak ser *and* weak nore, partly because autism is characterized by language delays and social awkwardness—

essentially anti-dominant characteristics (where strong ser or nore produce dominance; see Chapter 13). If weak ser and weak nore are responsible for language acquisition difficulties in autism, maybe people with strong ser or nore have superior linguistic skills. Whether autism can be treated by strengthening ser and nore during postnatal (i.e., after birth) development, and whether it can be treated later in life by the same means, is unclear. SRIs given after development have shown some efficacy. A possible experiment: give autistic individuals 1) an SRI only, 2) an NRI only, 3) both an SRI and an NRI. Another experiment (that will probably never be done): give one autistic identical twin ser and/or nore strengthening drugs during development, take the drugs away in adulthood, and then compare him with his never medicated twin. The bottom line is that autistic traits—such as low tolerance of stress; preservation of routine at all cost; that the illness may be precipitated by stressors; sensory sensitivity (though sometimes reduced sensitivity); paying attention to irrelevant details of objects; ADHD; depression; aggression; and sleep problems—all point to weak ser and possibly weak nore. An alternative hypothesis is that autism is caused by weak ser and/or strong nore

Impulse Control Disorders

These disorders may be caused by Big Three abnormalities interacting with hardwired circuits, and therefore are partially treatable with Big Three drugs. Inability to control anger may have two components: an intense feeling of anger itself, and the inability to prevent reaction to this feeling. As with drug and alcohol abuse, these disorders may be related to overt mental illnesses, such as ADHD (hypofrontality) and bipolar disorder (hypomania or mania). Weak ser and/or strong nore, accompanied by either weak or strong dop, may be the principal Big Three abnormalities.

Eating Disorders

I think these disorders are almost always accompanied by Big Three abnormalities, especially weak ser and/or strong nore. If self-esteem is partly encoded by strength of ser (see Chapter 7), then weak ser causing low self-esteem may play a critical role. Moreover, perhaps there is sometimes a relationship between weak ser and perceiving oneself as physically unattractive. As in drug and alcohol abuse, weak dop stimulus seeking may also play a role.

The eating disorders often coexist with other mental illnesses such as bipolar disorder, consistent with the hypothesis that ser tends to be weak and nore tends to be strong in both eating disorders and bipolar disorder.

Self-injurious behavior may also be characterized by weak ser and/or strong nore, and should be responsive to The Adjustment.

CHAPTER 11

EXPANDED DYSTHYMIA

Major Points

• **Over 50% of the population may be mildly depressed (expanded dysthymic) in that their quality of life could be made higher—possibly dramatically higher—by The Adjustment, allowing them to live up to their full potential.**

• **Describes the relationship between expanded dysthymia and 'searching' (i.e., continuously altering one's lifestyle to find contentedness), of which high achievement is a special case.**

• **Draws an analogy between poor vision (sightedness) and expanded dysthymia, both of which affect complex organs— the eye and the brain—and both of which are very common.**

Here I am expanding the concept of dysthymia, or mild long-term depression, to include a much broader array of individuals who generally haven't been considered to have anything wrong with them, but nonetheless have non-optimal Big Three strengths. Expanded dysthymia may also include many or all people with overt mental illnesses. The term is somewhat misleading because it refers here to more than just mood, but then again depression is known to affect Big Three traits other than just mood. I'm not suggesting that everyone with expanded dysthymia has an overt mental illness, just that their quality of life is not as high as it could be.

Expanded dysthymia results when any one of the Big Three— especially ser or nore—is too strong or too weak, and is worse if more than one of them is too strong or too weak. The further from optimal Big Three strengths a person is, the greater the magnitude of the dysthymia. So we can think of the expanded dysthymia circuits as a logical NOT for ser and nore (see Chapter 6), in that ser and nore are not both at mid-range, optimal strengths. One extreme possibility is that nearly 100% of the population is expanded dysthymic; another extreme is that fewer than 10% are—which is even lower than the percent diagnosed with overt mental illnesses in their lifetime. My estimate is that it includes over 50% of the population. And it is possible that, in spite of the potential side effects of existing Big Three drugs, over 50% of the population would experience higher quality of life if The Adjustment were performed properly on them with these drugs. Based on Big Three personality traits that I have observed, most expanded dysthymics have weak ser and/or strong nore; in fact, most of the population has weak ser and/or strong nore. Strong nore or strong ser are two special cases of expanded dysthymic types, and are perhaps the dysthymic types most likely to exhibit dominance (see Chapter 13).

There's a tendency to think that 'normal' or at least 'average' is bad, but maybe having average (optimal, mid-range) ser and nore strengths is amazing, though this may actually be quite uncommon. All people who have or previously had the overt mental illnesses previously mentioned may qualify as expanded dysthymic also, though not all dysthymics exhibit overt, *DSM-IV-TR* diagnosable mental illnesses. Ratey and Johnson (*Shadow Syndromes*) and Kramer (*Listening to Prozac*) point out that there exist so-called forme fruste disorders characterized by a few, possibly subtle versions of the symptoms—or perhaps no overt symptoms—of the full-blown mental illness. My point is that for expanded dysthymia a person can have *zero* conventional mental illness symptoms.

When The Adjustment works and corrects expanded dysthymia, I'm guessing it beats money, fame, power, prestige, or any combination thereof. If most dysthymics knew what they were missing, they'd be willing to fight for the treatment. A widespread belief is that there is no response to antidepressants unless someone is depressed, or more generally it is widely believed that there is no response to Big Three drugs unless someone is overtly mentally ill. I disagree: there is always a response when the Big Three are altered, including in the correction of expanded dysthymia.

High Achievement and Searching

The current theory hypothesizes that expanded dysthymia is so common because it motivates one to achieve, due to dissatisfaction with what one has. So an intraspecies (within the human race) evolutionary 'arms race' may have selected for high achievement, and therefore selected for large numbers of dysthymics. In this scenario, high achievement was selected for by evolution for at least two reasons: because the high achiever tends to possess both higher social status and greater physical resources such as possessions, leading to greater reproductive success. Perhaps the advent of civilization and living in very large groups intensified the arms race. In addition, human migration about the globe in the last 100,000 years may have selected for dysthymia to drive that migration—those who were happy got left behind. In other words, perhaps the human race used to be happier. So evolution cast us into this world, but only made some of us half-alive, since evolution does not practice utilitarianism—which is the principle of producing the greatest good for the greatest number of people—or even at all produce similar quality of life among different individuals. Some of us have wonderful lives, and others have miserable lives. So it can be viewed as an evolutionary engineering flaw, or consequence, that many of us have Big Three abnormalities. In summary, mental pathology, though not necessary for high achievement, often drives it.

If expanded dysthymia and high achievement are closely related, then maybe megalomania—which is a preoccupation with grandiose or extravagant things or actions—is the thought process that drives high achievement, because the person doesn't have normal emotional responses to normal stimuli. Perhaps necessary for megalomania: weak or nonexistent emotional responses to normal stimuli. A related idea is that if emotions are maxed out or very strong to normal stimuli, then seeking greater stimuli is unlikely. In other words, if a person has robust emotional responses to small stimuli that saturate at a certain point that is no lower than that which is evoked by large stimuli, they would have no motivation other than reason to pursue megalomaniacal goals. Megalomania may be more common in men than in women, and American culture may encourage it, for better or for worse. Along these lines, is expanded dysthymia overrepresented in the United States, due to dysthymic immigration? Not only does the United States attract high achievers, but also the culture reinforces this behavior. It would be interesting to compare the prevalence of expanded dysthymia in different countries. Maybe expanded dysthymia is also overrepresented among academics—a type of high achiever—versus the general population. I think being super strong in one or more of the Big Three—where being super strong produces subtypes of expanded dysthymia—makes high achievement more likely, because this indicates dominance. However, dysthymia in and of itself may produce a type of dominance (see Chapter 13).

If many expanded dysthymics are workaholics, they probably act this way because for them, the rewards of working may be about as good as life gets. So dysthymia may drive high achievement in part by 'keeping the feet to the fire', with the dysthymic person feeling compelled to work super hard. On the other hand, some dysthymics seem to have lower than average ambition.

Expanded dysthymia could drive high achievement but so could euthymia or a strong brain reward system—they both can and probably do. So even without dysthymia it would probably still be human nature to strive for something better, to be ambitious.

There may also be a fine line between high achievement and no achievement. In other words, paradoxically, as dysthymia increases among different people, high achievement can increase while ability to function decreases—cases in point: famous artists, certain politicians and leaders such as Abraham Lincoln, certain businessmen such as Howard Hughes. If expanded dysthymia turns out to affect most of the population, including all socioeconomic groups, and we medicated nearly every one of these people and wiped out most of the dysthymia, we may then be less ambitious as a society—perhaps at this point in history that may not be such a bad thing. I think most individuals within the population should be similarly dysfunctional in Big Three abnormalities. So maybe many people are dysthymic enough that they barely function, but not more so, producing high ambition.

If *super* non-optimalities of ser and nore produce low achievement, since the person is not able to function, perhaps the graph of achievement versus ser and/or nore optimality has an inverted U-shaped curve (see Figure 3), with somewhat of a non-optimality producing highest achievement. Such a curve would also predict the existence of pairs of data points—the intersections of horizontal lines—for which achievement is the same but the member of the pair with greater non-optimality has a lower quality of life than the other member. If one can get equivalent performance or achievement with greater quality of life, then one should always choose greater quality of life.

Perhaps high achievement is actually a special case of 'searching' caused by expanded dysthymia. Searching, or more specifically high achievement, does not always follow from dysthymia, but dysthymia perhaps makes it more likely. Searching means that one is continuously altering one's lifestyle—significant other, job, hobbies, place of residence, etc.—to find contentedness, which one never quite achieves. Like the special case of high achievement, searching may have been selected for by evolution because it led to greater reproductive success. Dysthymia may drive searching but do other mild forms of mental illness?

The thought process that may accompany searching is what I call 'false attribution'. This means blaming the way the world is—or at least one's situation in the world—for one's unhappiness instead of blaming one's own brain. Along these lines, some people think that the current modern environment is at least partly responsible for making them unhappy. I take a more cynical stance: they would have been just as unhappy (dysthymic) if they had lived prior to civilization.

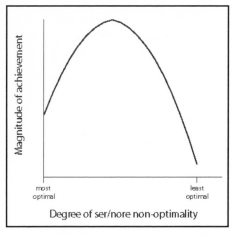

Figure 3

A concept related to searching is what I term 'the stationary test', which consists of asking whether one can remain content or even function without frequently having major changes in one's lifestyle. This test can be thought of as pass/fail, or instead one can think of it as having intermediate answers, such as that one is able to function *somewhat* without major changes in lifestyle.

Searching may not in all cases be caused by expanded dysthymia, since psychological environmental adaptation, in other words burnout or situational depression, may be another cause, and such adaptation may be more intense for people with strong dop, as in Cloninger's 'novelty seeking' dop trait, discussed in the next chapter. But whether due to expanded dysthymia or strong dop adaptation, the constant or at least recurrent need for fundamental changes in one's lifestyle may reflect underlying Big Three strength pathology.

Relationship to Dominance

In people with expanded dysthymia, the brain may in some ways be shut down. Shutting down of the brain—or deadening of Big Three traits, see Chapter 7—due to Big Three strength abnormalities, is closely related to shutting down of the brain with dominance (see Chapter 13). More generally, quality of life is not just a matter of mood, but also how the brain responds to the world, and this is affected by Big Three functional traits.

The ways in which different expanded dysthymics perceive the world probably vary greatly, though all or nearly all dysthymics may have one trait in common: lack of, or at least diminished, positive perception of and reaction to the world. Maybe deadening of mood and positive emotional responses—'the glow goes away'—is the universal characteristic of expanded dysthymia and at least most types of dominance. In other words, there may be similar aspects to perception across all cases of dysthymia.

Losses and Gains

Because the Big Three affect many functional traits (see Chapter 7) that may exist as continua, adjusting ser and/or nore with drugs to treat expanded dysthymia can also be seen as producing an exchange of traits, namely a loss/diminishment of some and a gain/enhancement of others. We can call such an exchange 'lossful' if it produces a net decrease in quality of life, 'gainful' if it produces a net increase in quality of life, or 'neutral' if there is no net change. If performed properly, The Adjustment should always produce a gainful exchange, though it may not always be perceived this way because personality and behavioral habits are set up to engage in positive activities optimized for the former Big Three traits. In other words, the person may be more familiar with what they lost than with what they gained.

In some people there could be the opposite bias in that there's a positive novelty effect to The Adjustment that would wear off in time, though others may find such novelty disagreeable. In either case, letting a given person assess the sign of their own exchange may be unreliable. If we could anticipate and then tell them what the gains and losses are, then maybe they could better assess them. So the quality of an exchange may not be apparent immediately but only after one has lived with it for a while. We can even define expanded dysthymia as including everyone who has—or would have—a gainful exchange to The Adjustment, which may include over 50% of the population. The further the Big Three are from optimal strengths in a given person, the greater the magnitude of the gainful exchange produced by The Adjustment. So The Adjustment has a diminishing return—in other words, a weaker effect—the closer the Big Three are to their optimal, mid-range strengths to begin with. And the concept of gainful and lossful exchanges partly depends on whether there are optimal ranges for ser and nore strength, or instead whether there is an optimal point for each. Finally, Big Three strength adjustment possibly isn't the whole story with expanded dysthymia, as the hardwired brain circuitry probably differs from person to person. That said, adjusting ser and/or nore in everyone will produce some effect that should increase or decrease the magnitude of the dysthymia.

Maybe when The Adjustment is performed on an expanded dysthymic person, he then has less of a specialized personality and is more so a generalist, in that he is more generally capable. In other words, he gains a broader range of skills and talents. If so, treating expanded dysthymia with The Adjustment may not harm society, and may in fact make it function better, possibly much better. However, perhaps it's a good thing for society that a given person may only be able to be adjusted so much.

An Analogy

One can draw an analogy between poor vision (sightedness) and expanded dysthymia; both: 1) are very common; 2) can be improved by medical intervention; 3) may not be present at birth and can have various ages of onset; 4) seem like they would be selected against by evolution, but may in some cases be selected for; 5) may be more common now due to evolutionarily recent changes in the environment, or changes in evolutionary selective pressure; 6) are mediated by complex organs—the eye and the brain—though the brain is obviously more complex; 7) are special cases of the many things that can go wrong with the eye and the brain, though sightedness and expanded dysthymia are by far the most common things that do go wrong with these organs; 8) are of critical importance to the well being and survival of the individual; 9) have a degree of dysfunction that may be a continuum; 10) are similar in that the worse it is the more likely the person is to know that something is wrong, but he may not fully appreciate that something was wrong until it is fixed; and 11) may have a clear, optimal solution, though adjusting ser/nore may be a matter of personal taste in terms of gainful and lossful exchanges.

Special Types

Now I'll provide some comments on four special types of expanded dysthymia: strong nore, strong ser, weak nore, and weak ser. For each of these four types, there may be no single personality type—there are many, just as there are many weak ser mental illnesses. All four of these types may differ from one another in their percentages of males and females, as women, on average, appear to be stronger in nore and weaker in ser than men. By extrapolation from the propranolol study mentioned in Chapter 9, maybe someone with super strong nore detects sadness better in others because he evolved, through natural selection, to recognize discontent in others and thereby lead the way to subversion of authority, though many people may identify with the underdog subverting authority. Super strong ser people may be aloof and compassionate, whereas super strong nore people may be empathetic, at least in most cases for both types of people. I'm not sure if there's a substantial market for ser weakening drugs, because strong ser is so rare, though many ser weakening drugs already exist. A related point is that there have probably been few cases in which a super strong ser person was given an SRI (which is clearly pathological, as in My Case Study), though there probably have been a lot more cases in which a super strong nore person has been given an NRI, which for them should be pathological. Since the SRIs have unveiled a broad array of people who may be weak in ser (as Michael Norden points out in *Beyond Prozac*), might there also be a broad array of people who are weak in nore? Finally, some weak ser people are cheerful and some are not—does this represent hardwired differences in circuitry? Are both types nonetheless expanded dysthymic?

CHAPTER 12

PERSONALITY

Major Points

• The vast differences in personality between people are primarily due to the interaction of hardwired brain circuits and Big Three strengths.

• Describes eminent psychiatric researcher C. Robert Cloninger's Big Three personality model, as well as the popular Enneagram model.

• Strength of ser is related to one's sense of identity.

• Artists have strong nore and weak ser systems—as is the case with many people—and this may explain the increased prevalence of bipolar disorder in artists.

• Describes a personality type exemplified by Clint Eastwood, Bill Belichick, and the author.

What makes one person enjoy working in a flower shop and another enjoy driving a dump truck? People are vastly different—why? In general, men are vastly different from women, and there's huge variability within each sex, too. Behavior is certainly vastly different, both between and within sexes. And due to Big Three differences, people are not only vastly different from one another but may also, as stated earlier, experience vastly different quality of life, and actually perceive the world very differently. The current theory hypothesizes that these personality differences are due to the interaction of Big Three strength differences and hardwired circuitry differences. In other words, two people can have the same Big Three strengths and still have vastly different personalities due to hardwired circuitry differences. I see these personality differences as largely genetic and largely invariant throughout life, particularly throughout adulthood. Indeed, personality may be a reliable indirect measure of Big Three strengths, particularly if hardwired differences are considered. Therefore, personality traits should be considered when prescribing drugs for the various mental illnesses, as well as for expanded dysthymia.

So, as described in Chapter 7, altering the strengths of the Big Three with drugs should alter personality traits, a phenomenon that Peter Kramer discusses in his landmark book, *Listening to Prozac*. Moreover, I think personality is intimately intertwined with mental illness, since most personality traits are affected by the Big Three, and the Big Three also intimately affect mental illness. Personality and mental illness are intimately related since they may both be produced by the same Big Three brain circuits.

Cloninger's Big Three Model

About twenty years ago, eminent psychiatric researcher C. Robert Cloninger created a personality model to explain the roles of the Big Three neurotransmitters in affecting behavior—though, unlike in The Triangle (see Chapter 5), Cloninger believed that the strengths of the Big Three are independent of each other, and that the Big Three presumably act on independent circuits. To ser he ascribed the role of "harm avoidance", which means ser causes the individual to act more boldly when faced with threatening or otherwise stressful situations. To nore he ascribed the role of "reward dependence", which means nore causes the individual to seek praise or acknowledgement from others. To dop he ascribed the role of "novelty seeking", which means dop causes the individual to seek new types of stimuli.

I think Cloninger is correct about the Big Three affecting these three traits, but I also think the Big Three interact in these roles, and as stated in Chapter 7, affect other traits as well. And as mentioned in Chapter 3, Cloninger's three traits may represent a form of pattern recognition mediated by the Big Three and their circuits that shapes behavior. In other words, the Big Three and their respective circuits allow the individual to recognize situations in the world relevant to harm avoidance, reward dependence, and novelty.

In spite of the obvious importance of Cloninger's ideas to psychiatry, I'm not sure Cloninger himself appreciated the full implications of his personality model, particularly the concept that the Big Three do more than just affect mood, and that the Big Three may be affecting personality traits in addition to the ones in his model. In one sense—especially when combined with the current theory—Cloninger's model may render all types of mental illnesses 'personality disorders', where abnormal strengths of the Big Three predispose one to or cause these illnesses.

In support of Cloninger's model, it has been shown experimentally that adjusting ser affects the harm avoidance trait. And perhaps being strong in nore causes a type of depression that is transiently relieved in a reward dependent manner, by acknowledgement from others.

I propose two variations on Cloninger's model that may make it more accurate: 1) both weak ser and strong ser may produce harm avoidance (to use the term very loosely), the latter because dominant individuals do not tend to recklessly endanger themselves; 2) both weak dop and strong dop may produce novelty seeking, the former because people with hypofrontality/ADHD tend to seek stimulation.

In considering the implications of Cloninger's model, there are several reasons why Big Three blood, urine, or cerebrospinal fluid (CSF) level studies, mainly carried out since the 1980s, haven't been too useful for treating mental illness: 1) before Cloninger's model it was not widely hypothesized that the Big Three affect personality; 2) personality is more complex than in Cloninger's model; 3) no one knows if there's a relationship between personality (or the levels themselves) and mental illness (treatment). So in other words, there may be very important information contained in level studies, if they really do indicate Big Three strength in most cases, as this information is relevant to performing The Adjustment with and without the presence of overt mental illness, but no one could confirm the validity of the blood, urine, or CSF data with an assessment of personality...possibly until the current theory.

The Enneagram Model

The popular Enneagram personality model, described most eloquently by Don Riso in his various books, is also relevant to understanding the relationship between the Big Three and personality. Despite its merits, the Enneagram, and perhaps other personality models, suffer from the same weaknesses as the disease models of the *DSM-IV-TR*: 1) failure to identify certain personality types, 2) unidentified subtypes within a type, and 3) incomplete descriptions of the existing types. So the Enneagram probably doesn't describe everyone well. For example, maybe people who aren't expanded dysthymic—who have mid-range, optimal strengths of the Big Three—don't have clear Enneagram personality types at all. But in its favor, the Enneagram personality types blend into one another, just as the mental illnesses blend into one another, and for most people the Enneagram provides a pretty good description.

What follows is not meant to be an exhaustive description of all Enneagram personality types, but instead mentions each one and subsequently elaborates upon a few of these types. Type 1: The Reformer (weak ser and possibly strong nore), Type 2: The Helper (weak ser and strong nore), Type 3: The Motivator (weak ser and strong nore), Type 4: The Individualist (weak ser and strong nore),

Type 5: The Thinker (weak ser), Type 6: The Loyalist (weak ser and medium nore), Type 7: The Enthusiast (weak ser and strong nore), Type 8: The Leader (either strong ser or strong nore), and Type 9: The Peacemaker (weak ser and medium nore).

In other words, most personality types—and perhaps most of the population—have weak ser and/or strong nore. In addition, most of the types, except 8 and possibly 7, have weak or medium dop, which is to some degree consistent with The Triangle (see Chapter 5). Note: adjacent numbers on the Enneagram blend into one another. Here are some famous examples of each type: mixtures of 1 and 2 (Andy Rooney, Oprah Winfrey), mixtures of 2 and 3 (Bill and Hillary Clinton, Michael Jordan, Tiger Woods), mixtures of 3 and 4 (Lance Armstrong, Pete Sampras, Andre Agassi, Arnold Schwarzenegger, John Kerry), mixture of 4 and 5 (Albert Einstein), mixtures of 5 and 6 (Stephen Hawking, Bill Gates), mixture of 6 and 7 (possibly Joan Rivers), mixtures of 7 and 8 (Donald Trump, George Steinbrenner, Hugh Hefner), mixtures of 8 and 9 (Ronald Reagan, Colin Powell, Shaquille O'Neal), mixture of 9 and 1 (possibly Nelson Mandela). The Enneagram also affords transitions—mixed personalities—between certain non-adjacent numbers. For example, the following people may be mixtures of 4 and 7: Robert Duvall, Tommy Lee Jones, Mark Cuban, Mick Jagger, Tom Green, and Mickey Rourke.

Maybe a tendency to view oneself in terms of how others regard one is related to one's sense of identity, and this may be related to the philosophical concept of weltschmerz ('world pain'). Enneagram types 2-4 can be described as lacking a strong sense of identity and having strong reward dependence. So a weak sense of identity may be encoded by weak ser and strong nore both interacting with particular hardwired circuits. While I was hypomanic on Zoloft and during bright light therapy, where both treatments may boost ser, I seemed to be more aware of myself.

The stereotypical artistic personality, in which the individual is sensitive, emotional, slightly depressed, and creative, is represented by the Enneagram type 4 personality—mixtures of types 3 and 4, or types 4 and 5—and has strong nore and weak ser. Artists also have acute senses, due to this high nore/ser ratio. Might they also have strong dop, where according to Cloninger's model, the desire for creativity could represent a type of novelty seeking? However, strong dop probably deadens the emotions, so it is unlikely to exist in most artists. Nonetheless, as discussed in the next chapter, strong nore may bestow a type of dominance, or at least prominence, much like strong ser, since many artists have achieved prominence and are widely revered. Weak ser and strong nore may explain the slightly depressive trait, and can be viewed as a form of expanded dysthymia (see Chapter 11). For these reasons, artists may in many cases have low self-esteem. On the other hand, this neurotransmitter array may give artists a strong capacity for mood to brighten when good things happen and a greater capacity for love—which may be related to the reward dependence characteristic of nore. And creativity, if not related to strong dop, may be a complex form of emotional expression, or can be stimulated by mania or hypomania in the course of typical bipolar disorder (see Chapter 10).

The following famous people may be or may have been artistic in both temperament and Big Three array (in alphabetical order): Woody Allen, Drew Barrymore, Warren Beatty, Halle Berry, Bono, Jim Carrey, Kurt Cobain, Sheryl Crow, Tom Cruise, James Dean, Robert DeNiro, Robert Downey Jr., Michael Jackson, Kay Jamison, Scarlett Johansson, Stephen King, John Lennon, Jim Morrison, Joaquin Phoenix, Winona Ryder, Kevin Spacey, Steven Spielberg, Martha Stewart, Meryl Streep, and Steven Tyler. Kay Jamison, the eminent writer and psychiatric researcher, has gathered evidence that bipolar disorder is more common in artists than in the general population, and I think this is correct. However, the more general hypothesis is that the prevalence of (typical) bipolar disorder in artists is a special case of a more general phenomenon in that nearly all artists have strong or super strong nore.

The Enneagram also describes a prototypical hypomanic personality type—a mixture of types 7 and 8—who I think may be or may have been super strong in nore and dop, weak in ser (in alphabetical order): Alexander the Great, Muhammad Ali, Charles Barkley, Napoleon Bonaparte, George Custer, Jon Gruden, Rudy Guiliani, Hulk Hogan, Don King, Jack Nicholson, George Patton, Teddy Roosevelt, Lawrence Taylor, Ted Turner, Jesse Ventura, Mike Wallace, and Angus Young. Although this is not the classic 'alpha' personality type—which involves strong ser—it may nonetheless be the most common (typical) form of dominance (see Chapter 13). Note: I don't know if this personality type is necessarily more common in men than in women, especially since I believe men tend to be stronger in ser and weaker in nore than women. However, it could be that in our society, men of this personality type tend to become more prominent than women of this type.

The final personality type that I'll discuss does not fit well with the Enneagram model, though it is most closely related to the type 8 personality. This is what I call the atypical dominant individual, exemplified by Clint Eastwood, Bill Belichick, and myself. This type has super strong ser and dop, and weak nore. Eastwood and especially Belichick may not exhibit atypical bipolar disorder like myself, but they do at least exhibit atypical hypomania, in that they are very high in energy and very productive. Such a person will tend to be: masculine, somewhat asexual, aloof, usually skinny from lack of a strong appetite, not inclined to laugh or smile much, not easily excited, harm avoidant, interested in justice, poor at tolerating the cold, adept at explosive movements, deadened in senses and emotions (except for compassion), and somewhat low in mood. Since strong ser may be related to harm avoidance, it may cause preoccupation with one's own mortality—I experienced this more so while super strong in ser from Zoloft—and one can see it in some of Clint's movies, such as *Unforgiven*, though the effect may be confounded with standard depression; perhaps we weren't meant to ponder our own mortality excessively. This type may represent the classic alpha personality type, due to strong ser, though it may be very uncommon (atypical). Note: I believe this personality type is more common in men than in women, since I believe men tend to be stronger in ser and weaker in nore than women.

On a more general note: are people skilled at identifying Big Three characteristics in others, since this may be important for social interaction? I think that the super strong ser person is a natural psychologist, since understanding people is critical for achieving and maintaining power. And I don't think most of our government and big business leaders are super strong in ser, partly because ser represents atypical dominance. Finally, I think physical appearance—especially facial structure and expressions—correlates with personality type (and Big Three strength array), and if so this is relevant to mental health treatment.

CHAPTER 13

DOMINANCE AND LEADERSHIP

Major Points

• **Strong ser, nore, and dop may all correlate with dominance, consistent with underlying Big Three strength pathology. In this scheme, strong nore represents typical (most common) dominance and strong ser represents atypical (least common) dominance.**

• **Alternatively, dominance may be most likely when the individual has mid-range ser and nore strengths, and is therefore mentally healthiest and happiest.**

One can think of human dominance in terms of an expansion of the usual definition of dominance in animals that live in groups with pecking orders, known as dominance hierarchies. As with expanded dysthymia, I speak of human dominance in a more general sense. It is partly related to intelligence, and also related to sensory-emotional deadening. One could measure human dominance in terms of money, fame, prestige, or power, though none of these measures may provide a clear indication. Society may indeed be largely arranged in terms of hierarchical organizations, such as governments and corporations—consistent with different degrees of dominance in different people—but this may have little to do with human nature, and simply is a logical way to structure large organizations.

Undoubtedly, the picture of dominance in humans is very complex. According to the scientific literature, which includes animal studies, strong ser, nore, or dop all correlate with dominance. Moreover, weak dop, if it produces stimulus seeking, may also produce dominance. Dominance may also have something to do with hardwired circuits, and may in general reflect underlying Big Three pathology. Perhaps any phenotype (i.e., behavioral characteristic)—possibly including traits based on *low* Big Three strengths—in which there is dissatisfaction with small rewards promotes dominance, which can be viewed as a type of high achievement (see Chapter 11). Alternatively, dominance may be most likely when an individual has mid-range ser and nore strengths and is euthymic, and perhaps the other dysthymic Big Three dominant neurotransmitter types evolved to mimic such true dominance. In other words, the dysthymic dominant types represent 'sham' or 'false' dominance, because in reality they are not as dominant as the euthymic individual.

The two most common Big Three dominant types are strong nore (which I call 'typical' dominance because it's so common) and strong ser (atypical dominance, which is quite rare). Both types tend to have strong dop as well, as described in The Triangle (see Chapter 5). So people exhibiting the most common form of dominance may actually have a below average strength of ser. Both typical and atypical dominance—especially if accompanied by strong dop—may produce emotional deadening, and atypical dominance should produce sensory deadening as well, due to a high ser/nore ratio. Sensory and emotional deadening may correlate with dominance because the dominant individual has the most environmental stress and should only react to the most salient sensory and emotional stimuli. In other words, it's stressful being at the top, for a variety of reasons, including the possibility that others are plotting against one, and the dominant one must be careful not to waste opportunities by reacting to unimportant things.

It makes sense that dominance can be characterized by expanded dysthymia/shutting down of the brain, as the dominant one should not be satisfied with the status quo, and should always be seeking to improve his situation. After all, this type of thinking may be what made him dominant in the first place, and also maintains his dominance.

An alternative way of viewing dominance, mentioned at the start of this chapter, is that it's caused by euthymia rather than dysthymia, which, combined with the observation that expanded dysthymia may produce dominance, means just about any temperament can produce dominance. Moreover, intelligence may represent a type of dominance independent of neurochemical temperament, especially if the opposite is hypofrontality and low intelligence. Likewise, low intelligence may have evolved in a subset of humans to fulfill a submissive sociological niche, even though the marked expansion of the brain over the last several million years of evolution suggests that high intelligence was strongly selected for.

In Peter Kramer's latest book, *Against Depression*, he describes our widespread fascination with depressed individuals; perhaps recognition of depression, and our fascination with depression, is hardwired into the brain, since depression may be related to dominance, and recognition of dominance, including our selection of leaders, has probably been selected through evolution. Indeed, many leaders throughout history, if not overtly mentally ill in the conventional sense, exhibited characteristics bordering on pathology, which would probably qualify as expanded dysthymia. I'm not suggesting this justifies or fully explains their, in some cases, ruthless behavior, but it's part of the picture. Examples: Abraham Lincoln, Winston Churchill, Napoleon Bonaparte, Adolf Hitler, and perhaps Alexander the Great.

What is the relationship between ser and leadership, since strong ser may produce classical dominance? Is the ser system simply designed to allow a person to achieve and maintain power, possibly by finding out what other people want and delivering it? If ser bestows the trait of harm avoidance, how important is it for the future welfare of this planet that our leaders be strong in ser, since such leaders might instinctively avoid potential catastrophes? And if ser tends to inhibit aggression, and many leaders have weak ser and are aggressive, then isn't it dangerous for the world to have such leaders in power? I think having strong ser leaders is critical for the future welfare of the planet. This is just as important as understanding and affecting how power is structured and the dynamic forces that affect it. Similarly, it may be important for the human race to know that the super strong ser (atypical dominant) person can be compassionate and perhaps is designed for leadership, and possibly doesn't usurp power. It's important for us if this type has been in power throughout human history but is no longer.

Finally, it makes sense that dominance, and therefore strong dop or hypomania, should coexist with paranoia, regarding the suspicion that others are plotting against one. But paranoia may also produce submissiveness, as in schizophrenia, due to weak ser. From an evolutionary perspective, one can see how paranoia and delusions could be useful to produce submissiveness/low status or, instead, to maintain dominance; perhaps these traits help produce both personality niches. More generally, perhaps some cases of mental illness were selected for to affect dominance or submissiveness, where depression alone can produce submissiveness.

CHAPTER 14

EVOLUTION

Major Points

- **Mental illness in humans may have been shaped by evolution for hundreds of thousands of years.**

- **The Big Three may exist to *produce* mental illness and thereby drive behavior.**

- **Evolution does not practice utilitarianism, which is the principle of producing the greatest good for the greatest number of people—it just shapes behavior without necessarily optimizing the conscious experience of the individual.**

I believe the overt mental illnesses and expanded dysthymia are not something new and specific to the 20th and 21st centuries, but have been around and shaped by evolution for hundreds of thousands of years, though this doesn't mean mental illness is not increasing in frequency and/or severity with recent increases in environmental stress. Some of these disorders may be present in other animal species, particularly other mammals, since many animals—perhaps all mammals, for example—have the Big Three. It seems probable that evolution would have weeded out most of the mild mental illnesses—along with the severe ones—if they weren't adaptive (that is, if they didn't improve survival and reproduction); but then again, poor eyesight hasn't been weeded out.

Why do the Big Three systems exist at all, from an evolutionary perspective? Their brain circuits could in principle operate in default states without Big Three input. Could it be that they exist to *produce* mental illness, especially depression or expanded dysthymia, to drive behavior? Of course, the Big Three affect many personality traits, and mental illnesses can be seen as special cases of personality traits. So the principal function of the Big Three could be to produce personality types that fit various sociological niches. In this scenario, maybe the evolutionary 'objective' for every person is dominance within their personality niche, making them the best at what they do, and thereby most effective at passing along their genes. In either case, evolution seems to have selected for weak ser and/or strong nore in terms of sheer numbers of people—other Big Three types are much more rare. But it did not weed out strong ser and/or weak nore—those alleles (the variants of a gene) are either less common or they are not less common but expressed in fewer people.

Maybe depression, or mental illness in general, is something hardwired into the brain—a depression circuit, related to the neural integrator hypothesis (see Chapter 2), that the Big Three turn on and off—selected for by evolution to produce behavior, especially searching, as described in Chapter 11. In order for such a circuit to be selected for, the depressive effect has to be either mild or transient—perhaps no more than a few months in duration—whether or not there's an external cause; otherwise the person just stays severely depressed and can't function again. More specifically, depression in particular, and mental illness in general, may only be selected for by evolution if it is: 1) caused by external events that the depressed person is aware of; 2) is reversible within a reasonable amount of time—these two points are necessary in order for the depressed person to learn from his experiences; or 3) if not 1 and 2, is constant (or seasonal) but mild, since unending severe depression would greatly impair survival and reproduction. Point 3 is strongly related to the concept of searching (see Chapter 11), and points 1 and 2 may also coexist with searching.

People who are depressed tend to choose other depressed people as their mates, a phenomenon called assortative mating, discussed by Raymond DePaulo in *Understanding Depression*. An idea related to assortative mating is that parents may harbor genes that are expressed in their offspring to make the offspring's personality more compatible with theirs.

Pleiotropy, which is the control by a single gene of several distinct and seemingly unrelated effects on the person, may also have affected the evolution of mental illness, and may be one of the reasons mental illnesses are so common. For example, each of the multiple genes that encode nore strength may affect mental health via the brain, as well as affecting the heart, and both of these functions could have simultaneously been shaped by evolution. In particular, if one of these nore genes improved the function of the heart dramatically (which is clearly a strongly positive effect) while also producing very mild depression (let's call this a weakly negative effect) due to its effects on the brain, that gene could have been selected for and preserved in the gene pool due to its more prominent effect on the heart, thereby preserving the mild depression.

So, via pleiotropy, mental illness traits may have co-evolved with other bodily traits such that the mental illness is overshadowed by the other traits that are being selected for, or vice versa, and the genes are then passed on. The existence of a systemic ser or nore level (see Chapter 4), which affects many bodily functions simultaneously, particularly many brain circuits, is consistent with this hypothesis. Also, mental illness itself could be selected for by producing benefits early in life while not producing them later in life, when the illness may get more severe. In addition, a particular mental illness in a particular environment could either be selected for or against, or be approximately neutral.

We can imagine four possible types of selection for (or against) mental illness in humans throughout their evolutionary history, though

I don't have a strong opinion as to which one is correct: 1) not prior to civilization and not since then, 2) not prior to civilization but since then, 3) prior to civilization but not since then, 4) both prior to civilization and since then. Indeed, selective pressure may be very different now than it was throughout much of evolutionary history because the environment (civilization) has changed so much, particularly in the last 100 years, though maybe this environmental difference is not as large as it seems to be. For example, in evolutionary history, loss (such as the death of a loved one) isn't a new type of stressor and other types of stressors may not be that different now.

Mental illness may never (including now) have been selected for, but accumulates now because it is not being strongly selected against—a genetic drift theory.

Finally, one might object to adjusting the Big Three with drugs because this alters one's nature or essence, but evolution created one's nature, and should one be beholden to evolution—a force that doesn't at all necessarily optimize quality of life—or instead have some choice in one's nature? In other words, evolution does not practice utilitarianism, which is the principle of producing the greatest good for the greatest number of people—it just shapes behavior without necessarily optimizing the quality of the conscious experience of the individual. Evolution doesn't care if you enjoy yourself, or even if you're miserable, as long as you perform—that is, engage in behaviors that pass along your genes. Of course, the way one feels and perceives the world can strongly influence behavior, and in fact, dysphoria can drive behavior that may be selected for. So evolution acts directly on behavior and indirectly on conscious and unconscious mental states that drive behavior.

CHAPTER 15

GENETICS

Major Points

• **Most of the genes that produce mental illness probably affect the Big Three systems, which are each multi-gene systems, and all or nearly all mental illnesses have at least a partial genetic basis.**

• **Specific genes have already been associated with particular mental illnesses, such as depression, bipolar disorder, and schizophrenia.**

• **Offspring probably aren't simply Big Three strength mixtures of their parents, consistent with widespread expanded dysthymia.**

I think most of the genes that produce mental illness affect the robustness of the Big Three systems, which are each multi-gene systems, and all or nearly all mental illnesses have at least a partial genetic basis. Many of these Big Three genes probably affect the postsynaptic circuitry, and their effects are not limited to neurons that possess Big Three external receptors. Even though there are undoubtedly many genes that affect the Big Three systems, it's not as if every gene necessarily does something unique to each system—there may be redundancy in that separate genes could effectively produce the same Big Three strength and phenotype (behavioral characteristic). And there may be master control genes that switch the development and/or activation of Big Three circuits on or off.

Specific alleles, which are the variants of a gene, such as those encoding the ser and nore reuptake transporters—the molecules that pump ser and nore out of the synapse—have already been associated with particular mental illnesses, such as depression. Many other mental illnesses, such as bipolar disorder and schizophrenia, have also been associated with particular genes. In such cases, there is a probabilistic association of the allele with mental illness in a large number of people, but for a particular person the given allele is probably neither necessary nor sufficient for the illness, consistent with Big Three strengths being encoded by multiple genes.

It will be interesting to see how the genetics of the Big Three play out: 1) Are offspring mixtures of their parents? In other words, do offspring simply possess a blending of their parents' Big Three systems?; 2) How are sex differences between parents and their offspring inherited?; 3) More generally, to what extent do offspring really resemble their parents? Regarding 2), keep in mind that the current theory hypothesizes that men tend to be stronger in ser and weaker in nore than women (see Chapter 7). So we could describe a man with strong ser and weak nore as having a theoretical 'female match' who represents a reversal of these strengths, namely weak ser and strong nore. If this man's female offspring inherited his Big Three genes, rather than his mate's Big Three genes, these offspring would be weak in a ser and strong in nore. And if his male offspring inherited his Big Three genes, these offspring would be, like him, strong in ser and weak in nore. In other words, in this scenario, genetic transmission of ser and nore genes is 'sign-preserving' between a parent and child of the same sex, whereas transmission is 'sign-reversing' between a parent and child of the opposite sex.

Furthermore, if nearly everyone is expanded dysthymic, then offspring probably aren't Big Three strength mixtures of their parents, and therefore aren't just mixtures of the alleles of the parents— otherwise, more people would be content. The most plausible hypothesis may be that there's a higher probability of the offspring resembling the parent(s) in both Big Three strengths and hardwired circuitry, though there's a chance, due to the presence of other alleles, that those offspring bear little resemblance to the parents.

CHAPTER 16

THE ROLE OF TALK THERAPY

Major Points

• **Several different schools of thought on talk therapy, also known as psychotherapy, emerged in the 20th century.**

• **Scientific studies have shown that some types of psychotherapy are effective in treating mental illness, especially when used in conjunction with medication.**

• **Psychotherapy may have its role transformed in a positive way in light of The Adjustment.**

The 20th century was a very exciting time for the field of psychiatry. With the emergence of Freudian psychoanalysis in the early part of the century, other schools of thought on talk therapy, also known as psychotherapy, soon followed. In the 1940s, the American Aaron T. Beck put forth cognitive therapy (also known as cognitive behavior therapy (CBT)), which focuses on correcting distortions in the patient's thinking that negatively impact his quality of life. By developing a more realistic and positive view of himself and his place in the world, the patient can have a more fulfilling life. In the 1950s, another American, Carl Rogers, put forth humanistic psychotherapy, which is based on a positive view of human nature and focuses on the patient developing a greater understanding of himself with the guidance of an empathetic therapist. Around this time, existential psychotherapy, put forth by Viktor Frankl and others, emerged out of existential philosophy, as another school of thought. It focuses upon trying to maintain a sense of meaning in life in spite of the many limitations of human existence, such as impending death. Another school of thought, called behavioral psychotherapy, emerged by the 1960s, and was put forth by B.F. Skinner and others. It focuses on modifying observable pathological behavior in the patient through such techniques as classical conditioning, which train the unwanted behavior away.

There is now ample scientific evidence that psychotherapy, especially cognitive therapy, is effective in treating overt mental illnesses, particularly when used in conjunction with psychiatric medication. Indeed, psychotherapy has been demonstrated to aid in the treatment of depression, bipolar disorder, schizophrenia, anxiety disorders, and others, and may in some cases be as effective as or more effective than medication, at least in the manner in which medication is currently being used. And similar to drug-based therapy, psychotherapy has been shown to have measurable effects on brain function, consistent with its efficacy in treating mental illness. It will be interesting to see how psychotherapy changes during the 21st century, as perhaps existing techniques could be modified and made even more effective, or perhaps entirely new schools of thought will emerge as well.

In spite of the merits of psychotherapy, psychiatric treatment may now be becoming increasingly drug-based—a biological psychiatry— particularly due to the widespread use of the SRIs such as Prozac, and it may seem that psychotherapy will play an increasingly smaller role in that treatment. After all, it's easier to take a pill once a day than it is to spend hours talking with a therapist. And the possibility that The Adjustment will render drug treatment far more effective, in a much wider array of people than previous drug treatment, may reinforce this trend. However, I don't think psychotherapy should be reduced in its role, even if The Adjustment does indeed deliver vastly better drug treatment than that which is typically produced by the current drug treatment. Rather, talk therapy should have its role *transformed* in light of The Adjustment, such that these two forms of treatment—drug and non-drug—complement one another more extensively and take on a more mutually beneficial relationship.

For example, as I mentioned in Chapter 11, The Adjustment can produce losses and gains in functional traits, but psychotherapy could facilitate the transition between the old self and the new self, helping the patient to adjust to these changes. And if The Adjustment, when it works fully, opens a new world of opportunity for the patient, of which he is not yet fully aware, the therapist could lead the proverbial kid to the candy store. On the other hand, if The Adjustment has a more limited effect in a particular patient, the therapist could help the patient cope with the reality that life is often less than ideal. Finally, since many people will probably be unwilling to try The Adjustment, for a variety of reasons, even if they suffer from moderate to severe mental illness, psychotherapy can by itself still provide invaluable help in such cases.

CHAPTER 17

NEW DIRECTIONS FOR IMPROVING PSYCHIATRY

Major Points

- **Brain scans and blood measures may allow for objective measurement of Big Three strengths and quality of life, which would greatly help in implementing The Adjustment.**

- **The neurotransmitter acetylcholine is very similar to the Big Three in its brain distribution and may also need to be at a mid-range strength for optimal mental health.**

- **Nore drugs are underused in psychiatry and are critical for implementing The Adjustment.**

Will psychiatry ever move beyond subjective assessments, in which the doctor simply observes the patient and then decides how to treat him? Affect, or more generally behavior, may only loosely correlate with mental illness, and our ability to assess behavior subjectively is limited and often unreliable. A more objective psychiatry might measure Big Three strengths—both baseline and responses to a drug—in a given person, not just from an interview and behavioral patterns, but also from a questionnaire (possibly a variation of Cloninger's Big Three questionnaire that is already being used for scientific research), a blood (plasma, serum, platelet) test, a saliva test, a urine test, a cerebrospinal fluid (CSF) test, a brain scan (PET, SPECT, MRI, EEG), Big Three drug challenge paradigms (which measure hormonal responses to Big Three drugs), genes, or perhaps some formula that combines these data. Measuring Big Three strengths objectively may be an essential step toward improving psychiatric treatment dramatically. Knowing the Big Three strengths would not only make it clearer how to adjust a given person, but also a cost-benefit analysis could be performed to decide whether to perform The Adjustment at all. For example, the presence of highly non-optimal Big Three strengths in a given person could render The Adjustment likely very beneficial to them, which could be weighed against the cost of potentially causing a 3+ year brain freeze. In addition, brain imaging measures of the average activation of certain brain areas may provide objective neural correlates of quality of life; in other words, a person's self-reported quality of life may be directly proportional to how much certain brain areas 'light up' in PET or MRI scans.

Here are a few notes on studies of brain imaging of the Big Three, using PET, SPECT, or MRI. Nearly all of these studies have focused upon the ser system, with very few data on the nore system. Most of the studies have focused upon the ser reuptake transporter, which is the molecule that is acted upon by the SRI drugs. Other studies have measured the brain distribution of the ser 5HT_2A receptor or the rate of ser brain synthesis, where both measures may be related to ser strength. So far, there are no brain imaging data on nore synthesis.

In terms of drug treatment, in the foreseeable future, when drugs are the principal treatment available for mental illness, will the distribution of Big Three receptor subtypes in the brain set the limits on the specificity of particular drugs? And how many receptor subtypes remain to be discovered? After all, scientists have already identified about a dozen different ser receptor subtypes, and there are multiple nore and dop receptor subtypes as well. Nonetheless, I hypothesize that there may be only a limited number of receptor subtypes that are relevant to the current theory, such as the ser 5HT_2A receptor.

Circuitry differences in intracellular properties could also affect drug specificity, and drugs that act on intracellular signaling cascades may also set specificity of treatment. Maybe 100 years from now, nanotechnology, or some other technology, will change the way drugs are delivered or develop another technique, like replacing or replicating neuronal circuits in the brain; or there may be a non-invasive device for stimulating specific circuits in the brain, which might be a variant of transcranial magnetic stimulation (TMS), a technique that is already being used to treat depression.

Improving the Current Theory

How can we go about creating a better model than the current theory? After all, it isn't so much that the ideas presented in this book are all necessarily correct, but rather that this type of reasoning will lead to a greater understanding of the brain and improved treatment in psychiatry. Everyone possesses the ability to reason, and applying such reasoning based on common sense and perhaps combined with information about how the brain and other parts of the body work, may lead to an improved psychiatry. Start with simple models—preferably those that present testable hypotheses—and modify or discard those models if they aren't consistent with the data. For example, one could take at face value that the SRIs really do selectively strengthen ser, that the NRIs selectively strengthen nore, that the atypical antipsychotics weaken ser and dop, that clonidine and the other alpha 2 adrenergic agonists weaken nore; and that there are systemic Big Three strengths coupled with hardwired circuitry differences. Then continue building a new model based on those premises.

Can abnormalities of one or more of the Big Three neuro-transmitter systems explain every type of mental illness? Probably not. What I've called 'Big Three traits' may also be affected by other brain transmitter systems, such as acetylcholine, histamine, GABA, glutamate, endogenous opioids, endogenous cannabinoids, and various other protein transmitters. Let's touch upon some of these other transmitter systems now.

Acetylcholine is most similar in its brain distribution to the Big Three, including having presynaptic cells in the brainstem that send connections throughout the brain, and its cortical circuits undoubtedly overlap with those of ser and nore, so it may be the additional transmitter most likely to affect Big Three traits and play a role in mental illness. Acetylcholine is also known to interact with ser and nore during sleep—possibly in an antagonistic manner—and its neurons fire action potentials consistently during sleep and inconsistently during waking. It also appears to affect vigilance. There are several acetylcholine level boosting drugs that are FDA approved to treat Alzheimer's disease, and it would be interesting to see if and how these drugs affect overt mental illnesses and expanded dysthymia. Perhaps, as for ser and nore, there is a single, systemic level of acetylcholine, and this transmitter system needs to be at a mid-range strength for optimal mental health.

Histaminergic neurons of the small brain region called the hypothalamus send connections to broad regions of the brain and fire action potentials actively during waking, though their function is not well understood. GABA, which may be the brain's principal inhibitory neurotransmitter in that it tends to quell neural activity, has already been shown to play an important role in the treatment of anxiety, as two classes of drugs, the barbiturates and the benzodiazepines, whose effects kick in immediately, are thought to act on GABA receptors. And drugs that affect glutamate, which may be the brain's principal excitatory neurotransmitter in that it tends to activate other neurons, have been shown, in a preliminary manner, to possess an antidepressant effect. GABA and glutamate undoubtedly affect circuits that overlap with those of the Big Three. And the prostaglandins, which may not act as neurotransmitters but rather as intracellular signaling molecules, may also affect mental health, as Michael Norden has pointed out in *Beyond Prozac*.

Keep in mind that with all the molecular changes that take place in mental illnesses and with their drug treatment, we must identify those changes that actually affect mental health—many may be dead ends, such as cellular 'housekeeping functions' that simply keep the neuron alive and healthy, having very little directly to do with mood, cognition, and other traits. As stated in Chapter 3, I believe that to affect mental health, a molecular or cellular process must affect neuronal electrical properties. However, affecting electrical properties is not sufficient to affect mental illness: the process must also affect the relevant circuits. But that includes a lot of processes, such as ion channels, structural aspects of neurons such as dendritic spines and axon growth, presynaptic vesicles, etc. Intracellular signaling cascades may only be relevant, at least in the short term, if they affect ion channels, which allow charged particles to flow in and out of neurons. Other molecular processes that affect the development of neurons may be shown to be relevant in the future.

Using Existing Drugs More Effectively

Pre-emptively adjusting the Big Three may prevent future mental illness in vulnerable individuals, but first we have to pre-emptively identify such individuals. Perhaps we could do so genetically or via a Big Three strength blood assessment. Moreover, being able to predict the optimal dose of a given drug for a given person would improve psychiatry tremendously.

Adjusting the strength of nore is critical for The Adjustment. Alpha or beta receptor activators and deactivators, besides clonidine and the other alpha 2 adrenergic agonists, may turn out to be useful nore adjusting drugs. Perhaps propranolol, a beta blocker, will turn out to be a clinically useful nore weakener. Indeed, there already exist a large number of alpha and beta nore activators and deactivators, and there are even alpha and beta receptor subtype specific activators and deactivators. First question: do all of these drugs enter the brain? Second, can nore postsynaptic deactivators treat typical bipolar disorder—and possibly strong nore expanded dysthymia—and if so which ones do? Third, can nore postsynaptic deactivators treat anxiety? Fourth, can nore postsynaptic activators (and deactivators) treat depression?

Finally, it would be great if the same psychiatric drugs were available in every country for a reasonable price, so that the practice of psychiatry could be similar and optimally effective throughout the world.

Creating New Drugs

I think drug development in the immediate future should focus upon creating more and possibly better Big Three drugs so that The Adjustment can be performed more effectively in a wider array of individuals. To do so, we can create drugs that are more neurotransmitter system/receptor subtype specific, though more people may then need to take a cocktail of drugs instead of a single drug to perform The Adjustment. Maybe a superior array of Big Three drugs would not only be more transmitter system/receptor subtype specific, but also be metabolized by the body in different, independent ways so there is no drug-drug breakdown interaction—this may not be possible, however. In addition, the multi-week delay in response to most Big Three drugs may be the single biggest obstacle to good psychiatric treatment. However, performing The Adjustment without a delay of at least many days may never be possible, due to intrinsic brain mechanisms, even with future drugs.

In general, drugs that affect external receptors on Big Three neurons (see Chapter 4) can: affect presynaptic transmitter release (increase or decrease it); affect transmitter reuptake (inhibit or enhance it); activate or deactivate postsynaptic circuits; affect breakdown of the transmitter (such as via the molecule monoamine oxidase (MAO), which breaks down the Big Three); or affect intracellular processes. By all of these mechanisms the circuitry may be affected by a drug. Potential new Big Three drugs could include: more ser presynaptic autoreceptor activators/deactivators that affect transmitter release; more ser reuptake enhancers, analogous to tianeptine; nore reuptake enhancers, also analogous to tianeptine; ser postsynaptic 5HT_2A receptor activators; ser postsynaptic 5HT_2A receptor deactivators, analogous to cyproheptadine; those that create more of or catalyze the MAO enzyme; reversible MAO inhibitors (which are already used outside the United States); and possibly those that affect synthesis of ser or nore. Some of the above drugs already exist and others are being synthesized and studied, partly by the drug companies. Maybe some types of new nore drugs would affect the brain without affecting the heart. And, as mentioned, perhaps the drug companies should develop a greater number of selective ser deactivators, similar to cyproheptadine, but there may not be a large market for these drugs since few people may have strong ser.

Why are there few dop strengtheners, such as Wellbutrin, on the United States market—especially if their effects kick in immediately? Maybe the reason is that, as Samuel Barondes points out in *Better than Prozac*, some dop strengthening drugs may mimic the effects of cocaine, producing an addictive high.

Is the NRI reboxetine—not currently available in the United States—superior to other NRIs in terms of its side effect profile?

A dual nore/dop deactivator, analogous to the atypical antipsychotics (ser/dop deactivators), could be a landmark drug for typical bipolar disorder, other overt mental illnesses, and expanded dysthymia. This could be a large market drug.

Molecular research may reveal other ways, and develop other drugs, to affect the circuits that the Big Three act upon. If there are other means, including drugs, to access the Big Three circuitry, these other means may kick in faster than in several weeks or may be less reversible in their effects, though reversibility is probably a good thing. Maybe a drug that nourishes Big Three neurons—if this is possible—would be effective and lasting in its effects. And maybe a drug could be created that mimics the antidepressant effect of exercise. Likewise, maybe a drug could be created that mimics the effects of ECT. Such drugs would be most useful if exercise and ECT affect the brain in ways other than the mechanisms of existing Big Three drugs. And if we could create a drug that stopped psychological adaptation to positive environmental stimuli—that is, stopped burnout—it might sell better than Prozac!

If side effects can be minimized, Big Three drug use may become as common as vitamin use—the SRIs already nearly make this a reality—and ser/nore receptor specific activators and deactivators may move the field of psychiatry further in this direction.

The Drug Companies

There's a tendency by the public to vilify the drug companies, whose for profit motive doesn't often align with utilitarianism, but those companies created and reliably supply drugs that have saved millions of lives. If drug companies follow a for profit motive, maybe this is not that far from utilitarianism in one regard: first very general, large market share drugs are produced, then smaller niche drugs are produced, though these smaller niche drugs generate less revenue. However, I think drug companies would prefer to replace a large market drug (after its patent expires) with another large market drug as long as they are allowed to do so. Moreover, some of their marketing practices, including pricing, are clearly questionable. Since a free market produces this type of questionable behavior, the drug companies need to be regulated by a strong, objective FDA. One could even argue that the FDA, or some other federally funded organization, should develop psychiatric drugs—or sponsor their development—since the effects of mental illness greatly cost the government in lost wage taxes and disability payments.

Alternatively, perhaps the patent duration for psychiatric drugs should be extended to encourage financially riskier or smaller market share drugs to be produced. Indeed, since there is a very high cost for a drug company to bring a new drug to market in the United States—at least 100 million dollars, and maybe closer to one billion dollars—companies are now forced to produce drugs that they are quite confident will serve a fairly large market, such as drugs with very general mechanisms of action, like ser/nore dual reuptake inhibiting antidepressants.

CHAPTER 18

CLOSING THOUGHTS

Major Points

• **If The Adjustment works with the existing drugs, we could now have an enthusiastic revolution in which a large fraction of the population gives it a try, and the overtly mentally ill get much more effective treatment.**

• **The treatment of expanded dysthymia via The Adjustment may not only enrich people's lives but also make society function better, possibly much better.**

• **Whereas evolution may have created expanded dysthymia and the overt mental illnesses, it also rendered the brain, and life itself, potentially glorious, when there are mid-range Big Three strengths.**

Psychiatry is poised to have a lasting and profound effect on a large fraction of the population not previously considered for drug treatment—who have expanded dysthymia—while also providing much more effective treatment for the overtly mentally ill. If The Adjustment indeed works with the existing drugs, we could now have an enthusiastic revolution like the California gold rush, the race to the moon, the 1960s experimentation with illegal drugs, the dot.com boom, or, on a more cynical note, an arms race (to enhance various types of performance, as Peter Kramer has pointed out). In the least, psychiatry may become even more mainstream and destigmatized than it already is—not that psychiatric treatment has to be medicinal to be destigmatized, but rather that improvement of that treatment gives the field more credibility. Moreover, a greater understanding and recognition of the variants of mental illness, particularly the nearly ubiquitous mild forms, destigmatizes their treatment. On the research side of things, perhaps there should now be a race to map out the pharmacology of mental health and happiness. One could say this about all fields of medicine, but perhaps the Big Three drugs are more important for quality of life than most other non-psychiatric drugs. The bottom line is that the use of psychiatric drugs may become destigmatized to the level of vitamin use or, like my earlier analogy, eyeglasses. And perhaps acknowledging that mental illnesses, including expanded dysthymia, are biochemical disorders amenable to Big Three drug intervention further destigmatizes psychiatric treatment.

Do psychiatrists and researchers dislike the 'chemical imbalance' theories of mental illness, or variants of those theories, because they don't believe them, or because if such theories are true, they fear that this may in some ways trivialize what they do? After all, the current theory can be thought of as a variant of the chemical imbalance theories of mental illness from the 1960s and 1970s. However, it is not just balance of the strengths of ser and nore that is important, because the two cases of both ser and nore being weak or both ser and nore being strong each represent balance that is simultaneously pathological. Rather, the current theory hypothesizes that only when ser and nore have similar, mid-range strengths do they produce high quality of life. Moreover, dop can deviate significantly from a mid-range strength and perhaps be non-pathological.

It's actually still unclear to me whether all people with overt mental illness would benefit from The Adjustment—perhaps in some cases their ser and nore strengths are normal but dysfunctional. And perhaps the effects of The Adjustment, in addition to the potential brain freeze, are not always safe. Perhaps for some people The

Adjustment could have a catastrophic effect, analogous to the stress overload that causes some congenitally blind people to kill themselves when they gain sight later in life. However, I have trouble believing that many people would find The Adjustment so negatively disruptive, or even negative at all.

Effects of The Adjustment on Society

What about the effects of The Adjustment on society? For example, if everyone with expanded dysthymia was medicated and no longer sensed injustice in the world—and they were the only ones who previously sensed injustice, a premise that is almost certainly false—would injustice still exist, and what would this do to society? Arguing that we shouldn't adjust anyone with a severe mental illness because doing so may harm society is like arguing that we shouldn't treat toothaches for the same reason. However, the benefits of treating mild mental illness, and especially expanded dysthymia, are more debatable—doing so may clearly benefit the individual, but might it also harm society? I believe that society would actually function better—possibly much better—without mild mental illness or expanded dysthymia, though this may depend on how one defines societal functioning. For example, without expanded dysthymia there may be less of a collective effort to reform the world, since such adjusted individuals might lose other virtuous traits. However, perhaps a line should be drawn when functioning stops—then the individual should definitely be treated—though I suppose it could be argued that society could still function even if a substantial fraction of its individuals don't; but it seems ridiculous to argue that we should therefore deny them treatment. Moreover, perhaps the existing society is actually a direct reflection of widespread mental pathology, and if most of that pathology were eliminated, the world, including most human interactions, would be far healthier.

Nonetheless, given the potentially diverse experiences of The Adjustment among different people—some may like it and some may not—one could make the following two arguments for the benefit of society: 1) Maybe some people should be forced to be adjusted when they don't want to be for the betterment of society and possibly for their benefit as well, since they may later be jailed. For example, this might be done if there was a biological—perhaps a Big Three— abnormality that 100% of the time predicted violent criminal behavior and could be pre-emptively treated. 2) On the other hand, maybe some people should be denied The Adjustment if it was known that doing so would, on the whole, eliminate more traits that benefit society than enhance traits that do—a net decrease in societal benefit. Both 1) and especially 2), if enforced, may decrease quality of life for the individual, though if The Adjustment was performed in 1) it should almost always improve quality of life. In either case, an individual's right to be medicated—though this requires a professional health care provider's approval—and right *not* to be medicated, are both, to my knowledge, currently intact in nearly all cases in the United States.

Maybe the human race actually can't handle the society/ environment it has created without changing itself, possibly pharmacologically. Moreover, with The Adjustment, it's a lot easier to pharmacologically change one's perception of the world than it is to change the world itself. People who want to change the world and don't think they can be content unless it's changed might first want to try changing themselves. I'm not suggesting that there aren't important aspects of the world that should be changed, but rather that a powerful component in one's perception of the state of the world lies in the functional chemistry of one's own brain.

Final Thoughts

The Big Three drugs aren't soma from *Brave New World*, which was the 'opiate for the masses' in Aldous Huxley's famous novel. Soma controlled people, whereas these drugs stop one from being controlled by expanded dysthymia, which evolution created. Moreover, soma was intoxicating and these drugs are not. On the other hand, soma may be similar to these drugs in that it likewise simply relieved unhappiness. In addition, because expanded dysthymia affects so many people and is probably readily treatable in most, the Big Three drugs could potentially be used to control people by limiting their supply. Nonetheless, the treatment of expanded dysthymia and the overt mental illnesses represents, in my opinion, one of the few breakthroughs or innovations of civilization that has unequivocally improved quality of life. Contrarily, one could argue that eliminating expanded dysthymia could represent a fad, the novelty of which would wear off—something that could be tasted once, rather like visiting Paris in the spring or perhaps even having a single episode of major depression, to make a more well rounded person, to make life fuller. I don't think so, however—I believe it really does represent a sustained higher quality of life that is much more fundamental than a 'cosmetic' change, and therefore it won't be a passing fad.

The effectiveness of The Adjustment in treating nearly all types of overt mental illness, as well as improving the quality of life of expanded dysthymics, can be thought of as analogous to the central limit theorem of mathematical statistics, in that a wide variety of conditions converge on a single solution.

There are several stages of recovery from a mental illness (and perhaps any illness): 1) survival—the will to live, 2) functioning—taking care of oneself and providing for oneself if appropriate, and 3) contentment. With standard psychiatric drug treatment that does not employ the current theory, many people only reach stage 2, and some remain in stage 1. So there's a huge range of experience between being suicidal and being truly content, between death and being fully alive, and even between functioning and being fully alive; one might say 'as the brain was intended to be'. Evolution may have created expanded dysthymia, but it also rendered the brain, and life itself, potentially glorious, when there are mid-range Big Three strengths.

If expanded dysthymia is both as common and as treatable—with the existing drugs—as I think it is, and if we indeed pursue treatment of it on an international scale, then it's the end of the world as we know it, and I feel fine.

GLOSSARY

5HT_2A receptor: One of the many subtypes of brain ser receptors; I hypothesize that it is the only (or at least principal) ser postsynaptic receptor subtype relevant to treating mental illness.

acetylcholine: A neurotransmitter that is similar in its brain distribution to the Big Three and that may also be important for mental health. Has been implicated in learning and memory, including Alzheimer's disease. Also acts at the junction between nerves and muscles of the body.

action potential: An electrical wave that travels along the axon of a neuron, and is critical for transmitting information within and outside the brain.

acute: 1) Lasting a short period of time. 2) Very sensitive.

acute stress disorder: A post-traumatic stress disorder that occurs immediately or soon after a traumatic event.

The Adjustment: My term for a method of using pharmaceutical drugs to adjust ser and nore (and possibly dop) closer to mid-range, optimal strengths, and thereby improve quality of life for the individual.

agonist: A molecule, such as a neurotransmitter or drug, that activates a receptor.

agoraphobia: Fear of open or public places, which usually results in fear of leaving one's home.

alleles: The different varieties of a gene.

alpha 2 adrenergic agonists: Drugs that may weaken brain nore; or more specifically, may lower the brain level of nore, and possibly lower the level of nore in the rest of the body such as the heart.

alpha blockers: Drugs that may weaken brain nore by deactivating nore alpha receptors; also affect the heart.

American Psychiatric Association: A medical specialty society recognized worldwide, consisting of over 35,000 United States and international member physicians, most of whom are psychiatrists.

amygdala: An almond-shaped group of neurons in the anterior part of the temporal lobe of the brain that plays an important role in motivation and emotional behavior.

AND: My term for a system that requires that two or more components be intact in order for the system to function properly.

anorgasmia: Inability to achieve sexual orgasm.

antagonist: A molecule, such as a drug, that inactivates a receptor.

antidepressant: A drug designed to terminate depression.

antipsychotic: A drug designed to terminate psychosis (i.e., hallucinations and/or delusions). The older versions of these drugs are called typical antipsychotics, and the newer versions are called atypical antipsychotics. The typical antipsychotics deactivate dopamine receptors (and also may deactivate serotonin receptors, such as the 5HT_2A receptor), and the atypical antipsychotics deactivate dopamine and serotonin receptors (including the 5HT_2A receptor).

antisocial personality disorder: A personality disorder characterized by long-term antisocial behavior and violation of the law and the rights of others.

anxiety: A state of uneasiness or apprehension.

arrhythmia: A medical condition characterized by irregular heart-beat.

attention deficit hyperactivity disorder (ADHD): A mental illness, which usually first appears in childhood, that is characterized by inability to concentrate and hyperactivity.

atypical bipolar disorder: My term for a rare subtype of bipolar disorder that has underlying strong dop and ser, and weak nore.

atypical depression: Depression that is characterized primarily by oversleeping and overeating. I think it may be caused by weak ser and strong nore.

autism: A mental illness or developmental disorder with childhood onset that is characterized by marked deficits in communication and social interaction, preoccupation with fantasy, language impairment, and abnormal behavior.

autonomic nervous system: The part of the nervous system that regulates involuntary action, as of the intestines, heart, and glands, and that is divided into the sympathetic nervous system and the parasympathetic nervous system.

autoreceptor: A 'self' receptor; i.e., a receptor that receives neurotransmitter input from the same neuron that releases the neurotransmitter.

avoidant personality disorder: A personality disorder characterized by pervasive social inhibition, feelings of inadequacy, and hypersensitivity to negative evaluation.

axon: The tubelike portion of a neuron that generally transmits action potentials toward a synapse with another neuron or a muscle fiber.

basal ganglia: Large groups of neurons at the base of the brain involved principally in movement control.

beta blockers: Drugs that may weaken brain nore by deactivating nore beta receptors; also affect the heart.

Big Three: A term that Samuel Barondes and I have independently used to signify the neurotransmitters serotonin (ser), norepinephrine (nore), and dopamine (dop).

biogenic amines: Another name for the Big Three, as well as other brain chemicals, such as histamine, with a characteristic amine molecular structure.

biological: Concerning living things.

bipolar disorder (also known as manic-depressive illness): A mental illness characterized by episodes of mania or hypomania, that for nearly all bipolar persons is also characterized by episodes of depression.

bipolar I disorder: A subtype of bipolar disorder that is characterized by episodes of full-blown mania, and these episodes are in most cases interspersed with episodes of depression.

bipolar II disorder: A subtype of bipolar disorder that is characterized by episodes of hypomania, and these episodes are in most cases interspersed with episodes of depression; usually the depression is predominant.

block (a receptor): To deactivate a receptor with a molecule such as a drug.

borderline personality disorder: A personality disorder characterized by a long-standing pattern of instability in interpersonal relationships, behavior, mood, and self-image that can interfere with social or occupational functioning or cause extreme emotional distress.

brainstem: The portion of the brain that connects the spinal cord to the cerebral cortex.

brain freeze: My term for the mild depression and cognitive deficits that occurred when I took too high a dose of Zyprexa.

bright light therapy: A method of sitting in front of a bright light on a regular basis in order to treat seasonal affective disorder (SAD).

catatonia: A state of rigidity or flexibility of the limbs, characterized by lack of movement.

cerebral cortex: The extensive, folded layers of neurons of the cerebral hemispheres, largely responsible for higher brain functions, including sensation, voluntary movement, thought, reasoning, and memory.

cerebrospinal fluid (CSF): The extracellular fluid that bathes the brain and spinal cord.

chromosome: A large, folded strand of DNA and associated proteins.

chronic: Lasting a long period of time.

circuit: A set of synaptically interconnected neurons in the brain that form a functional unit.

clinically relevant: Of practical importance to doctors.

cocaine: The street drug that acts as a dop reuptake inhibitor, and thereby is a strengthener of dop. It may also strengthen nore in the short term, but I think it's addictive 'high' is produced solely by short-term dop boosting.

cognition: Thinking and reasoning.

congenital: Present at birth.

continuum: Existing on a range or a scale.

convergence: Connected from many to one.

corollary: A deduction or inference.

cortical: Relating to the cerebral cortex.

critical period: A window of opportunity during brain development in which a skill or function, such as language, can be acquired.

CSF: see **cerebrospinal fluid**.

D2 receptor: One of several subtypes of dop receptors; it may be the only (or at least principal) dop receptor subtype relevant to treating mental illness. It is also the site of action of some addictive drugs.

delusion: A false belief that is maintained in spite of clear evidence to the contrary.

dendrite: One of the principal synaptic receiving areas on a neuron; a single neuron usually has many dendrites.

dependent personality disorder: A personality disorder character-ized by pervasive and excessive need to be taken care of.

depression: A mental illness characterized by low or despondent mood, negative thinking, lack of interest in usual activities, sleep disturbance, and eating disturbance. Also known as major depression, clinical depression, and unipolar depression.

diurnal: Within a day.

divergence: Connected from one to many.

DNA (deoxyribonucleic acid): Molecule that forms the building blocks of genetic information in the cell.

dominance: Related to the relative position of an individual in a social hierarchy or pecking order, especially the highest position in that hierarchy.

dop (dopamine): One of the Big Three neurotransmitters; I think it plays a less important role in mental illness than ser and nore.

***DSM-IV-TR*:** The standard mental illness diagnostic text of the American Psychiatric Association.

dysfunction: Lack of proper functioning.

dysthymia: A mental illness characterized by long-term, mild depression.

eating disorder: Any of various psychological disorders, such as anorexia nervosa or bulimia, that involve insufficient or excessive food intake or digestion.

ECT (electroconvulsive therapy): Electrical stimulation of the brain that is used to treat mental illnesses, principally depression.

EEG (electroencephalography): A method for measuring electrical activity on the scalp that reflects the electrical activity of the brain.

electrical: Concerning the movement of charged particles.

endogenous: Originating from within the body; genetic or long-term environmentally influenced.

evolution: Change in the genetic composition of a population during successive generations, as a result of natural selection acting on the genetic variation among individuals, and sometimes resulting in the development of new species.

exogenous: Originating from outside the body; includes factors such as the seasons, drugs, stress, and possibly other recent environmental conditions such as sleep deprivation.

expanded dysthymia: My term that expands upon the usual definition of mild long-term depression to include a much larger fraction (perhaps over 50%) of the population who generally have not been considered to have anything wrong with them, but nonetheless have lower than possible quality of life due to non-mid-range Big Three strengths.

extracellular: Outside the cell (or neuron), or on the outer surface of the cell in the case of extracellular receptors.

FDA (Food and Drug Administration): The United States federal agency that regulates the pharmaceutical industry, among other duties.

flux: My term for a state of continuous mild depression produced by rapid (daily, weekly, or even monthly) changes in the types and dosages of Big Three drugs.

GABA: The brain's principal inhibitory neurotransmitter, in that it tends to decrease electrical activity in neurons.

gene: A particular sequence of DNA that, for most genes, encodes a protein.

generalized anxiety disorder: A long-term disorder characterized by persistent anxiety and such symptoms as tension, sweating, trembling, light-headedness, or irritability.

genetics: The science of heredity.

glutamate: The brain's principal excitatory neurotransmitter, in that it tends to increase electrical activity in neurons.

hallucination: A false sensation.

hardwired: My term for circuits in the brain whose characteristics are largely genetically determined and are not changeable.

histrionic personality disorder: A personality disorder characterized by excessive emotionality and attention-seeking behavior.

homeostasis: The ability of the body to maintain internal equilibrium by adjusting its physiological processes.

hypervigilance: The condition of maintaining an abnormally intense awareness of environmental stimuli.

hypofrontality: Decreased functioning of prefrontal cortex, resulting in inattention and impulsiveness.

hypomania: A milder version of mania characterized by elevated or irritable mood, racing thoughts, grandiose ideation, hyperactivity, and distractibility, without accompanying psychosis.

hypothalamic-pituitary-adrenal (HPA) axis: A group of related bodily structures that regulate responses to stress.

hypothalamus: A group of neurons that lies below the thalamus and regulates bodily temperature, certain metabolic processes, and other autonomic activities.

hypothesis: A tentative explanation for an observation, phenomenon, or scientific problem that can be tested by further investigation.

impulse control disorders: A family of disorders, such as substance abuse, pathological gambling, and explosive anger, characterized by a tendency to gratify an immediate desire or impulse, regardless of the consequences to oneself or to others.

impulsiveness: The trait of acting on impulse rather than on careful thought.

inherited: Passed genetically from parents to offspring.

interneuron: A 'local' neuron that synaptically connects neighboring neurons.

intracellular drug: My term for a drug that acts inside of neurons, rather than on their external receptors.

intracellular signaling cascade: My term for a series of chemical reactions that take place inside a neuron in response to a signal such as a drug or neurotransmitter; in many cases initiated by a drug or neurotransmitter binding to an external receptor.

ion channel: A molecule that allows charged particles (ions) to enter and/or leave neurons.

isomorphic: Literally, 'same form'. Here it means that the neural representation of a sensory stimulus in the brain takes the same form as the stimulus itself.

limbic system: A group of interconnected deep brain structures involved in smell, emotion, motivation, behavior, memory, and various autonomic functions.

linear system: A system in which the whole is equal to the sum of its parts.

LSD (lysergic acid diethylamide): The hallucinogenic street drug that I hypothesize to be a deactivator or weak activator of the ser

5HT_2A receptor.

major depression: A formal name for depression.

mammals: A class of warm-blooded vertebrate animals that give birth to live young; includes humans, monkeys, and rodents.

mania: A condition characterized by markedly elevated or irritable mood, racing thoughts, grandiose ideation, hyperactivity, and distractibility, often with accompanying psychosis.

manic-depressive illness: see **bipolar disorder**.

megalomania: A preoccupation with grandiose or extravagant things or actions.

metabolize: To engage bodily processes in breaking down more complex molecules into simpler molecules, such as in the inactivation of drugs.

mixed mood: A condition in which someone exhibits both manic (or hypomanic) and depressed symptoms simultaneously.

molecule: An interconnected group of atoms that has distinct chemical properties.

mood: A baseline state of how one feels, whereas emotions are alterations produced by stimuli, such as sensory perceptions or memories, and are superimposed upon mood.

mood stabilizer: A drug that diminishes the magnitude and/or frequency of manic (or hypomanic) and depressive episodes in persons with bipolar disorder.

MRI (magnetic resonance imaging): A noninvasive diagnostic technique that produces computerized images of internal body tissues.

narcissistic personality disorder: A personality disorder characterized by excessive love or admiration of oneself, and extreme disregard for the feelings of others.

neural integrator hypothesis: My term for a circuit or group of circuits in the brain that is acted upon by the Big Three and controls a number of Big Three traits simultaneously, such as mood, emotion, sensory acuity, and others.

neuron: A cell in the nervous system that is capable of conducting electrical signals, and usually consists of a cell body, multiple dendrites, and a single axon, and is synaptically connected with other cells, within or outside the brain.

neurophysiology: The branch of neuroscience that studies the chemical properties of neurons, including their electrical properties.

neuroscience: The branch of science that studies the nervous system, including the brain.

neurotransmitter: A signaling molecule that is used for synaptic communication between neurons. It is typically released into the synapse by a neuron and binds to external receptors on the same or other neurons.

niche: 1) The function or position of an organism within an ecological community. 2) A special area of demand.

nonlinear system: A system in which the whole is not equal to the sum of its parts.

nore (norepinephrine): One of the Big Three neurotransmitters; relative to other neurotransmitters, I think it and ser play the most important roles in mental illness.

NREM (non-rapid eye movement) sleep: A recurring sleep state during which rapid eye movements do not occur and dreaming does not occur or is less vivid; accounts for about 75% of normal sleep time.

NRIs (nore reuptake inhibitors): Drugs that boost the level of nore in the brain. Include some of the tricyclic antidepressants, reboxetine, and Strattera.

object recognition: The ability to recognize familiar objects; a type of pattern recognition.

obsessive-compulsive disorder (OCD): A mental illness in which the person is beset with obsessions (recurrent thoughts) or compulsions (strong impulses to act) or both, and suffers extreme anxiety or depression if he or she fails to think the obsessive thoughts or perform the compelling acts.

obsessive-compulsive personality disorder: A personality disorder characterized by a preoccupation with orderliness, perfectionism, and mental and interpersonal control.

OR: My term for a system that requires that only one of two or more components be intact in order for the system to function properly.

overt mental illnesses: My term for the mental illnesses listed in the *DSM-IV-TR*.

panic attack: The sudden onset of intense anxiety, characterized by feelings of intense fear and accompanied by palpitations, shortness of breath, sweating, and trembling.

panic disorder: A disorder characterized by recurrent panic attacks and usually resulting in the development of one or more phobias, such as agoraphobia. It can be associated with a specific situational trigger.

parallel processing: The simultaneous processing of multiple types of information by multiple brain circuits.

paranoia: Extreme, irrational distrust of others.

paranoid personality disorder: A personality disorder characterized by consistent extreme and irrational distrust of others.

pattern recognition: The ability to recognize familiar patterns of stimuli, such as objects.

perception: The manner in which one experiences the world, including through the five senses.

peripheral nervous system: The part of the vertebrate nervous system constituting the nerves outside the central nervous system and including the cranial nerves, spinal nerves, and the autonomic nervous system.

permissive hypothesis: Theory that weak ser permits induction of full-blown mania in bipolar persons.

personality disorders: A group of disorders in which patterns of perceiving, relating to, and thinking about oneself and one's environment interfere with the long-term functioning of the individual, often manifested in deviant behavior and lifestyle.

PET (positron emission tomography): A noninvasive diagnostic technique that produces computerized images of internal body tissues.

pharmaceutical: A legal drug that is used to treat medical illnesses.

pharmacology: The science of drugs, including their composition, uses, and effects.

phenotype: The observable physical or biochemical characteristics of an organism, as determined by both genetic makeup and environmental influences.

placebo: A pill containing no active drug.

plasticity: The ability of the brain to change itself, usually in response to inputs.

pleiotropy: The control by a single gene of several distinct and seemingly unrelated phenotypic effects.

postsynaptic: Literally, 'after the synapse'. Related to receiving input from the presynaptic neuron.

Post-traumatic stress disorder (PTSD): A disorder affecting some individuals who have experienced or witnessed profoundly traumatic events, such as torture, murder, rape, or wartime combat, characterized by recurrent flashbacks of the traumatic event, nightmares, irritability, anxiety, fatigue, forgetfulness, and social withdrawal.

prefrontal cortex: Anterior portion of the cerebral cortex that is involved in cognition, emotion, and short-term memory.

presynaptic: Literally, 'before the synapse'. Related to sending input to the postsynaptic neuron.

proteins: Molecular chains of amino acids, with distinct chemical properties, that play a critical role in cellular function.

psychiatry: The branch of medicine that deals with the diagnosis, treatment, and prevention of mental illnesses.

psychology: The science that deals with mental processes and behavior.

psychophysics: The branch of psychology aimed at experimentally measuring properties of sensory perception.

psychosis: A mental condition characterized by hallucinations and/or delusions and/or thought disorder; occurs during some cases of schizophrenia, mania, and depression.

rapid (mood) cycling: Bipolar disorder that is characterized by four or more episodes of mania, hypomania, mixed mood, or depression within a 12 month period.

receptor: A cellular molecule that is capable of binding and responding to a signaling molecule such as a neurotransmitter or drug.

reinforcement of behavior: A positive or negative stimulus that strengthens or weakens the behavior that produced it.

rejection sensitivity: A trait of being extremely sensitive to social or interpersonal slights.

REM sleep: A stage in the normal sleep cycle during which most dreams occur and the body undergoes marked changes including rapid eye movement, loss of reflexes, and increased pulse rate and brain activity.

SAD (seasonal affective disorder): A form of depression occurring during certain seasons of the year, usually wintertime.

safety factor: My term for when the synaptic level of a neurotransmitter exceeds the point of saturation for its receptor population by a certain amount.

schizoid personality disorder: A personality disorder characterized by a pervasive pattern of detachment from social relationships and a restricted range of expression of emotions.

schizophrenia: A mental illness characterized by so-called positive symptoms (hallucinations, delusions, disjointed thought patterns) as well as so-called negative symptoms (apathy, social withdrawal, poverty of thought).

schizotypal personality disorder: A personality disorder characterized by a pervasive pattern of social and interpersonal deficits, as well as cognitive or perceptual distortions and eccentricities of behavior.

searching: My term for continuously altering one's lifestyle—significant other, job, hobbies, place of residence, etc.—to find contentedness, which one never quite achieves.

ser (serotonin): One of the Big Three neurotransmitters; relative to other neurotransmitters, I think it and nore play the most important roles in mental illness.

serial processing: The sequential processing of information within a single brain circuit.

social phobia: Extreme, debilitating fear associated with situations in which one is potentially subject to criticism by others.

specific phobias: Disorders characterized by marked and persistent fear of specific objects or situations.

SPECT (single photon emission computed tomography): A noninvasive technique for imaging brain structures.

SRIs (ser reuptake inhibitors): Drugs that boost the level of ser in the brain. Examples include Prozac, Zoloft, Paxil, Lexapro, and Luvox.

strength (of the Big Three): My term which means the extracellular level of the neurotransmitter plus the sensitivity of the brain circuitry to that level.

synapse: The place at which an electrical signal (usually an action potential) passes from one neuron to another.

systemic: Throughout the body.

tardive dyskinesia: A potentially irreversible movement disorder, characterized by tics and other involuntary movements, that is sometimes caused by the typical antipsychotics.

thalamus: The mass of neurons that lies between the brainstem and cerebral cortex, that essentially serves as a relay for electrical information to and from the cerebral cortex.

threshold: The point that must be crossed to produce a given effect.

Tourette's syndrome: A disorder characterized by facial and other body tics, usually beginning in childhood and often accompanied by grunts and compulsive utterances, such as interjections and obscenities.

transmitter: My abbreviation for 'neurotransmitter'.

The Triangle: My term for the putative, long-term strength interactions that occur between the Big Three.

tricyclic antidepressants: A class of drugs that boost nore, where some of these drugs boost ser as well. The tricyclic NRIs are desipramine, nortriptyline, and protriptyline.

typical bipolar disorder: My term for a common subtype of bipolar disorder that has underlying strong dop and nore, and weak ser.

unipolar depression: A fancy term for depression that is not accompanied by additional episodes of mania, hypomania, or mixed mood states.

utilitarianism: The philosophical principle that one's actions should produce the greatest good for the greatest number of people.

weltschmerz: The philosophical principle of sorrow over the perceived present or future evils or woes of the world in general; sentimental pessimism.

REFERENCES

Chapter 1. A Brief History of Psychiatry

Samuel H Barondes, *Better than Prozac*, Oxford Univ Press, New York, NY, 2003.

Coppen A (1967) The biochemistry of affective disorders. Br J Psychiatry 113:1237-1264.

Janowsky DS, El-Yousef MK, Davis JM, Sekerke HJ (1972) A cholinergic-adrenergic hypothesis of mania and depression. Lancet 2:632-635.

Michael J Norden, *Beyond Prozac*, ReganBooks, New York, NY, 1995.

Schildkraut JJ (1965) The catecholamine hypothesis of affective disorders: a review of supporting evidence. Am J Psychiatry 122:509-522.

Siever LJ, Risch SC, Murphy DL (1981) Central cholinergic-adrenergic balance in the regulation of affective state. Psychiatry Res 5:108-109.

www.wikipedia.com

Chapter 2. My Case Study

Andy Behrman, *Electroboy*, Random House, New York, NY, 2002.

Chapter 3. General Characteristics of Brain Function
Sensory Systems

Bruce Alberts, Dennis Bray, Julian Lewis, Martin Raff, Keith Roberts, James D Watson, *Molecular Biology of the Cell, 3rd Edition*, Garland Publishing, New York, NY, 1994.

Felleman DJ, Van Essen DC (1991) Distributed hierarchical processing in the primate cerebral cortex. Cereb Cortex 1:1-47.

Information Processing

Eriksson PS, Perfilieva E, Bjork-Eriksson T, Alborn AM, Nordborg C, Peterson DA, Gage FH (1998) Neurogenesis in the adult human hippocampus. Nature Medicine 11:1313-1317.

Gage FH (2002) Neurogenesis in the adult brain (review paper). J Neurosci 22:612-613.

Steinmetz PN, Roy A, Fitzgerald PJ, Hsiao SS, Johnson KO, Niebur E (2000) Attention modulates synchronized neuronal firing in primate somatosensory cortex. Nature 404: 187-190.

Chapter 4. Enter the Big Three

Saturation of Ser and Nore, with a Safety Factor

Bjorvatn B, Gronli J, Hamre F, Sorensen E, Fiske E, Bjorkum AA, Portas CM, Ursin R (2002) Effects of sleep deprivation on extracellular serotonin in hippocampus and frontal cortex of the rat. Neuroscience 113:323-330.

Florin SM, Kuczenski R, Segal DS (1994) Regional extracellular norepinephrine responses to amphetamine and cocaine and effects of clonidine pretreatment. Brain Res 654:53-62.

Lena I, Parrot S, Deschaux O, Muffat-Joly S, Sauvinet V, Renaud B, Suaud-Chagny MF, Gottesmann C (2005) Variations in extracellular levels of dopamine, noradrenaline, glutamate, and aspartate across the sleep-wake cycle in the medial prefrontal cortex and nucleus accumbens of freely moving rats. J Neurosci Res 81:891-899.

Lopez-Rodriguez F, Wilson CL, Maidment NT, Poland RE, Engel J (2003) Total sleep deprivation increases extracellular serotonin in the rat hippocampus. Neuroscience 121:523-530.

Maisonneuve IM, Keller RW, Glick SD (1990) Similar effects of D-amphetamine and cocaine on extracellular dopamine levels in medial prefrontal cortex of rats. Brain Res 535:221-226.

Moghaddam B, Bunney BS (1989) Differential effect of cocaine on extracellular dopamine levels in rat medial prefrontal cortex and nucleus accumbens: comparison to amphetamine. Synapse 4:156-161.

Monti JM, Jantos H, Monti D, Alvarino F (2000) Dorsal raphe nucleus administration of 5-HT1A receptor agonist and antagonists: effect on rapid eye movement sleep in the rat. Sleep Res Online 3:29-34.

Nicolaidis S, Gerozissis K, Orosco M (2001) Variations of hypothalamic and cortical prostaglandins and monoamines reveal transitions in arousal states: microdialysis study in the rat. Rev Neurol (Paris) 157:S26-33.

Pan WH, Lai YJ, Chen NH (1995) Differential effects of chloral hydrate and pentobarbital sodium on a cocaine level and its catecholamine response in the medial prefrontal cortex: a comparison with conscious rats. J Neurochem 64:2653-2659.

Park SP (2002) In vivo microdialysis measures of extracellular norepinephrine in the rat amygdala during sleep-wakefulness. J Korean Med Sci 17:395-399.

Penalva RG, Lancel M, Flachskamm C, Reul JM, Holsboer F, Linthorst AC (2003) Effect of sleep and sleep deprivation on serotonergic neurotransmission in the hippocampus: a combined in vivo microdialysis/EEG study in rats. Eur J Neurosci 17:1896-1906.

Portas CM, Bjorvatn B, Ursin R (2000) Serotonin and the sleep/wake cycle: special emphasis on microdialysis studies. Prog Neurobiol 60:13-35.

Python A, Steimer T, de Saint Hilaire Z, Mikolajewski R, Nicolaidis S (2001) Extracellular serotonin variations during vigilance states in the preoptic area of rats: a microdialysis study. Brain Res 910:49-54.

Sakai K, Crochet S (2001) Differentiation of presumed serotonergic dorsal raphe neurons in relation to behavior and wake-sleep states. Neuroscience 104:1141-1155.

Shouse MN, Staba RJ, Saquib SF, Farber PR (2000) Monoamines and sleep: microdialysis findings in pons and amygdala. Brain Res 860:181-189.

Stecker RE, Thakkar MM, Porkka-Heiskanen T, Dauphin LJ, Bjorkum AA, McCarley RW (1999) Behavioral state-related changes of extracellular serotonin concentration in the pedunculopontine tegmental nucleus: a microdialysis study in freely moving animals. Sleep Res Online 2:21-27.

Zeitzer JM, Maidment NT, Behnke EJ, Ackerson LC, Fried I, Engel J Jr, Wilson CL (2002) Ultradian sleep-cycle variation of serotonin in the human lateral ventricle. Neurology 59:1272-1274.

Dysfunction and Stress
Aston-Jones G, Rajkowski J, Kubiak P, Alexinsky T (1994) Locus coeruleus neurons in monkey are selectively activated by attended cues in a vigilance task. J Neurosci 14:4467-4480.

Clayton EC, Rajkowski J, Cohen JD, Aston-Jones G (2004) Phasic activation of monkey locus ceruleus neurons by simple decisions in a forced-choice task. J Neurosci 24:9914-9920.

Dazzi L, Seu E, Cherchi G, Biggio G (2005) Chronic administration of the SSRI fluvoxamine markedly and selectively reduces the sensitivity of cortical serotonergic neurons to footshock stress. Eur Neuropsychopharmacol 15:283-290.

Dazzi L, Vignone V, Seu E, Ladu S, Vacca G, Biggio G (2002) Inhibition by venlafaxine of the increase in norepinephrine output in rat prefrontal cortex elicited by acute stress or by the anxiogenic drug FG 7142. J Psychopharmacol 16:125-131.

Hajos-Korcsok E, Robinson DD, Yu JH, Fitch CS, Walker E, Merchant KM (2003) Rapid habituation of hippocampal serotonin and norepinephrine release and anxiety-related behaviors, but not plasma corticosterone levels, to repeated footshock stress in rats. Pharmacol Biochem Behav 74:609-616.

Jordan S, Kramer GL, Zukas PK, Petty F (1994) Previous stress increases in vivo biogenic amine response to swim stress. Neurochem Res 19:1521-1525.

Maier SF, Watkins LR (2005) Stressor controllability and learned helplessness: the roles of the dorsal raphe nucleus, serotonin, and corticotropin-releasing factor. Neurosci Biobehav Rev 29:829-841.

Nakane H, Shimizu N, Hori T (1994) Stress-induced norepinephrine release in the rat prefrontal cortex measured by microdialysis. Am J Physiol 267:R1559-1566.

Petty F, Jordan S, Kramer GL, Zukas PK, Wu J (1997) Benzodiazepine prevention of swim stress-induced sensitization of cortical biogenic amines: an in vivo microdialysis study. Neurochem Res 22:1101-1104.

Usher M, Cohen JD, Servan-Schreiber D, Rajkowski J, Aston-Jones G (1999) The role of locus coeruleus in the regulation of cognitive performance. Science 283:549-554.

Walletschek H, Raab A (1982) Spontaneous activity of dorsal raphe neurons during defensive and offensive encounters in the tree-shrew. Physiol Behav 28:697-705.

Waterhouse BD, Devilbiss D, Seiple S, Markowitz R (2004) Sensorimotor-related discharge of simultaneously recorded, single neurons in the dorsal raphe nucleus of the awake, unrestrained rat. Brain Res 1000:183-191.

Zhang X, Kindel GH, Wulfert E, Hanin I (1995) Effects of immobilization stress on hippocampal monoamine release: modification by mivazerol, a new alpha 2-adrenoceptor agonist. Neuropharmacology 34:1661-1672.

Continua Versus Thresholds

Rapoport JL, Buchsbaum MS, Weingartner H, Zahn TP, Ludlow C, Mikkelsen EJ (1980) Dextroamphetamine. Its cognitive and behavioral effects in normal and hyperactive boys and normal men. Arch Gen Psychiatry 37:933-943.

Chapter 5. Big Three Strength Interactions: The Triangle

Amargos-Bosch M, Artigas F, Adell A (2005) Effects of acute olanzapine after sustained fluoxetine on extracellular monoamine levels in the rat medial prefrontal cortex. Eur J Pharmacol 516:235-238.

Devoto P, Flore G, Longu G, Pira L, Gessa GL (2003) Origin of extracellular dopamine from dopamine and noradrenaline neurons in the medial prefrontal and occipital cortex. Synapse 50:200-205.

Devoto P, Flore G, Vacca G, Pira L, Arca A, Casu MA, Pani L, Gessa GL (2003) Co-release of noradrenaline and dopamine from noradrenergic neurons in the cerebral cortex induced by clozapine, the prototype atypical antipsychotic. Psychopharmacol (Berl) 167:79-84.

Gobert A, Rivet JM, Audinot V, Newman-Tancredi A, Cistarelli L, Millan MJ (1998) Simultaneous quantification of serotonin, dopamine and noradrenaline levels in single frontal cortex dialysates of freely-moving rats reveals a complex pattern of reciprocal auto-and hetero-receptor-mediated control of release. Neurosci 84:413-429.

Page ME, Lucki I (2002) Effects of acute and chronic reboxetine treatment on stress-induced monoamine efflux in the rat frontal cortex. Neuropsychopharmacology 27:237-247.

Pan WH, Yang SY, Lin SK (2004) Neurochemical interaction between dopaminergic and noradrenergic neurons in the medial prefrontal cortex. Synapse 53:44-52.

Pudovkina OL, Cremers TI, Westerink BH (2003) Regulation of the release of serotonin in the dorsal raphe nucleus by alpha1 and alpha2 adrenoceptors. Synapse 50:77-82.

Sodero AO, Valdomero A, Cuadra GR, Ramirez OA, Orsingher OA (2004) Locus coeruleus activity in perinatally protein-deprived rats: effects of fluoxetine administration. Eur J Pharmacol 503:35-42.

Tanda G, Carboni E, Frau R, Di Chiara G (1994) Increase of extracellular dopamine in the prefrontal cortex: a trait of drugs with antidepressant potential? Psychopharmacology (Berl) 115:285-288.

Yoshino T, Nisijima K, Katoh S, Yui K, Nakamura M (2002) Tandospirone potentiates the fluoxetine-induced increases in extracellular dopamine via 5-HT(1A) receptors in the rat medial frontal cortex. Neurochem Int 40:355-360.

Chapter 6. Big Three Circuits

Castren E (2005) Is mood chemistry? (review) Nat Rev Neurosci 6:241-246.

Levels of Scale

Haynes J-D, Rees G (2006) Neuroimaging: Decoding mental states from brain activity in humans. Nat Rev Neurosci 7:523-534.

Stefansson et al. (2002) Neuregulin I and susceptibility to schizophrenia. Am J Hum Genet 71:877-892.

Straub et al. (2002) Genetic variation in the 6p22.3 gene DTNBPI, the human ortholog of the mouse dysbindin gene, is associated with schizophrenia. Am J Hum Genet 71:337-348.

Effects of Drugs

Baron BM, Ogden AM, Siegel BW, Stegeman J, Ursillo RC, Dudley MW (1988) Rapid down regulation of beta-adrenoceptors by co-administration of desipramine and fluoxetine. Eur J Pharmacol 154:125-134.

Circuit Modulation

Cryan JF, O'Leary OF, Jin SH, Friedland JC, Ouyang M, Hirsch BR, Page ME, Dalvi A, Thomas SA, Lucki I (2004) Norepinephrine-deficient mice lack responses to antidepressant drugs, including selective serotonin reuptake inhibitors. Proc Natl Acad Sci USA 101:8186-8191.

Mood Circuits

Liotti M, Mayberg HS (2001) The role of functional neuroimaging in the neuropsychology of depression. J Clin Exp Neuropsychol 23:121-136.

Chapter 7. Big Three Functions
Sensation

Segal NL, Topolski TD, Wilson SM, Brown KW, Araki L (1995) Twin analysis of odor identification and perception. Physiol Behav 57: 605-609.

Emotion

Harmer CJ, Perrett DI, Cowen PJ, Goodwin GM (2001) Administration of the beta-adrenoceptor blocker propranolol impairs the processing of facial expressions of sadness. Psychopharmacol (Berl) 154:383-389.

Sleep

Kayama Y, Koyama Y (2003) Control of sleep and wakefulness by brain-stem monoaminergic and cholinergic neurons. Acta Neurochir Suppl 87:3-6.

Morgane PJ, Stern WC (1975) The role of serotonin and norepinephrine in sleep-waking activity. Natl Inst Drug Abuse Res Monogr Ser 3:37-61.

Reynolds CF (1987) Sleep and affective disorders. A minireview. Psychiatr Clin North Am 10:583-591.

Movement

Juhlin-Dannfelt A (1983) beta-Adrenoceptor blockade and exercise: effects on endurance and physical training. Acta Med Scand Suppl 672:49-54.

Leibowitz SF, Brown O, Tretter JR, Kirschgessner A (1985) Norepinephrine, clonidine, and tricyclic antidepressants selectively stimulate carbohydrate ingestion through noradrenergic system of the paraventricular nucleus. Pharmacol Biochem Behav 23:541-550.

Seznec JC, Lepine JP, Pelissolo A (2003) Dimensional personality assessment of the members of the French junior national team of road cycling. Encephale 29:29-33.

Disease
Palm D, Lang K, Niggemann B, Drell TL, Masur K, Zaenker KS, Entschladen F (2006) The norepinephrine-driven metastasis development of PC-3 human prostate cancer cells in BALB/c nude mice is inhibited by beta-blockers. Int J Cancer 118:2744-2749.

John J Ratey, Catherine Johnson, *Shadow Syndromes*, Bantam Books, New York, NY, 1998, p.20.

Vazquez SM, Mladovan AG, Perez C, Bruzzone A, Baldi A, Luthy IA (2006) Human breast cell lines exhibit functional alpha(2)-adrenoceptors. Cancer Chemother Pharmacol 58:50-61.

Gender Differences and Sexual Preference
Nishizawa S, Benkelfat C, Young SN, Leyton M, Mzengeza S, de Montigny C, Blier P, Diksic M (1997) Differences between males and females in rates of serotonin synthesis in human brain. Proc Natl Acad Sci USA 94:5308-5313.

Miscellaneous Traits
Brown GL, Linnoila MI (1990) CSF serotonin metabolite (5-HIAA) studies in depression, impulsivity, and violence. J Clin Psychiatry 51:31-43.

Ozawa H, Chen CS, Watanabe H, Uematsu T (1977) Effect of clonidine on blood pressure, heart rate and body temperature in conscious rats. Jpn J Pharmacol 27:47-54.

Chapter 8. The Adjustment
Skrebuhhova-Malmros T, Allikmets L, Matto V (2001) Additive effect of clonidine and fluoxetine on apomorphine-induced aggressive behavior in adult male Wistar rats. Arch Med Res 32:193-196.

Chapter 9. Effects of Drugs
Lane RM (1998) SRI-induced extrapyramidal side-effects and akathisia: implications for treatment. J Psychopharmacol 12:192-214.

Tse WS, Bond AJ (2002) Serotonergic intervention affects both social dominance and affiliative behaviour. Psychopharmacology (Berl) 161:324-330.

Ser Strengtheners
Samuel H Barondes, *Better than Prozac*, Oxford Univ Press, New York, NY, 2003, p.16.

Ser Weakeners
Akhondzadeh S, Mohammadi MR, Amini-Nooshabadi H, Davari-Ashtiani R (1999) Cyproheptadine in treatment of chronic schizophrenia: a double-blind, placebo-controlled study. J Clin Pharm Ther 24:49-52.

Balsara JJ, Jadhav SA, Gaonkar RK, Gaikwad RV, Jadhav JH (2005) Effects of the antidepressant trazodone, a 5-HT 2A/2C receptor antagonist, on dopamine-dependent behaviors in rats. Psychopharmacol (Berl) 179:597-605.

Blackshear MA, Martin LL, Sanders-Bush E (1986) Adaptive changes in the 5-HT2 binding site after chronic administration of agonists and antagonists. Neuropharmacol 25:1267-1271.

Davis R, Whittington R, Bryson HM (1997) Nefazodone. A review of its pharmacology and clinical efficacy in the management of major depression. Drugs 53:608-636.

Feder R (1991) Reversal of antidepressant activity of fluoxetine by cyproheptadine in three patients. J Clin Psychiatry 52:163-164.

Greenway SE, Pack AT, Greenway FL (1995) Treatment of depression with cyproheptadine. Pharmacotherapy 15:357-360.

McCormick S, Olin J, Brotman AW (1990) Reversal of fluoxetine-induced anorgasmia by cyproheptadine in two patients. J Clin Psychiatry 51:383-384.

Offord SJ, Warwick RO (1984) Ketanserin alters [3H]serotonin uptake and release in rat hypothalamus. Eur J Pharmacol 104:379-382.

Pazzagli M, Giovannini MG, Pepeu G (1999) Trazodone increases extracellular serotonin levels in the frontal cortex of rats. Eur J Pharmacol 383:249-257.

Wagstaff AJ, Ormrod D, Spencer CM (2001) Tianeptine: a review of its use in depressive disorders. CNS Drugs 15:231-259.

Nore Weakeners
Alary P, Andersson JC (1988) Clonidine: prophylactic action in rapid cycling manic-depressive psychosis. Encephale 14:119-126.

Blum I, Atsmon A (1976) The possible role of beta-adrenergic and alpha-adrenergic antagonist sensitive systems in the brain in the mechanism of psychosis. Med Hypotheses 2:104-106.

Chou JC (1991) Recent advances in treatment of acute mania. J Clin Psychopharmacol 11:3-21.

Coulin K, Simon O, Emrich HM, von Zerssen D (1982) The EEG of patients with acute manic psychoses before, during and after treatment with high doses of d-propranolol and dl-propranolol (author's transl). Arch Psychiatr Nervenkr 231:323-331.

Diacicov S, Tudorache B (1990) Clonidine treatment in manic episodes. Rev Med Interna Neurol Psihiatr Neurochir Dermatovenerol Neurol Psihiatr Neurochir 35:29-32.

Flemenbaum A (1981) The use and abuse of clonidine as a psychopharmacological tool. Prog Clin Biol Res 68:209-215.

Giannini AJ, Pascarzi GA, Loiselle RH, Price WA, Giannini MC (1986) Comparison of clonidine and lithium in the treatment of mania. Am J Psychiatry 143:1608-1609.

Gowing LR, Farrell M, Ali RL, White JM (2002) Alpha2-adrenergic agonists in opioid withdrawal. Addiction 97:49-58.

Gresch PJ, Sved AF, Zigmond MJ, Finlay JM (1995) Local influence of endogenous norepinephrine on extracellular dopamine in rat medial prefrontal cortex. J Neurochem 65:111-116.

Hardy MC, Lecrubier Y, Widlocher D (1986) Efficacy of clonidine in 24 patients with acute mania. Am J Psychiatry 143:1450-1453.

Hardy-Bayle MC, Lecrubier Y, Lancrenon S, Laine J, Allilaire JF, Des Lauriers A (1989) Clonidine versus a placebo trial in manic disorder. Encephale 15:523-526.

Janicak PG, Sharma RP, Easton M, Comaty JE, Davis JM (1989) A double-blind, placebo-controlled trial of clonidine in the treatment of acute mania. Psychopharmacol Bull 25:243-245.

Jimerson DC, Post RM, Stoddard FJ, Gillin JC, Bunney WE (1980) Preliminary trial of the noradrenergic agonist clonidine in psychiatric patients. Biol Psychiatry 15:45-57.

Johnson JM (1984) Psychiatric uses of antiadrenergic and adrenergic blocking drugs. J Nerv Ment Dis 172:123-132.

Jouvent R, Baruch P, Simon P (1986) Manic episode after propranolol withdrawal. Am J Psychiatry 143:1633.

Jouvent R, Lecrubier Y, Puech AJ, Simon P, Widlocher D (1980) Antimanic effect of clonidine. Am J Psychiatry 137:1275-1276.

Kontaxakis V, Markianos M, Markidis M, Stefanis C (1989) Clonidine in the treatment of mixed bipolar disorder. Acta Psychiatr Scand 79:108-110.

Maguire J, Singh AN (1987) Clonidine. An effective anti-manic agent? Br J Psychiatry 150:863-864.

Mateo Y, Fernandez-Pastor B, Meana JJ (2001) Acute and chronic effects of desipramine and clorgyline on alpha(2)-adrenoceptors regulating noradrenergic transmission in the rat brain: a dual-probe microdialysis study. Br J Pharmacol 133:1362-1370.

Moller HJ, von Zerssen D, Emrich HM, Kissling W, Cording C, Schietsch HJ, Riedel E (1979) Action of d-propranolol in manic psychoses. Arch Psychiatr Nervenkr 227:301-317.

Peet M, Yates RA (1981) Beta-blockers in the treatment of neurological and psychiatric disorders. J Clin Hosp Pharm 6:155-171.

Pudovkina OL, Kawahara Y, de Vries J, Westerink BH (2001) The release of noradrenaline in the locus coeruleus and prefrontal cortex studied with dual-probe microdialysis. Brain Res 906:38-45.

Rackensperger W, Fritsch W, Schwarz D, Stutte KH, Zerssen D (1976) The effect of the beta-adrenergic blocking agent propranolol in mania (author's transl). Arch Psychiatr Nervenkr 222:223-243.

Robson RD, Antonaccio MJ, Saelens JK, Liebman J (1978) Antagonism by mianserin and classical alpha-adrenoceptor blocking drugs of some cardiovascular and behavioral effects of clonidine. Eur J Pharmacol 47:431-442.

Saper JR, Lake AE, Cantrell DT, Winner PK, White JR (2002) Chronic daily headache prophylaxis with tizanidine: a double-blind, placebo-controlled, multicenter outcome study. Headache 42:470-482.

Stoudemire A, Brown JT, Harris RT, Blessing-Feussner C, Roberts JH, Nichols JC, Houpt JL (1984) Propranolol and depression: a reevaluation based on a pilot clinical trial. Psychiatr Med 2:211-218.

Szabo B, Fritz T, Wedzony K (2001) Effects of imidazoline anti-hypertensive drugs on sympathetic tone and noradrenaline release in the prefrontal cortex. Br J Pharmacol 134:295-304.

Tudorache B, Diacicov S (1991) The effect of clonidine in the treatment of acute mania. Rom J Neurol Psychiatry 29:209-213.

Van Gaalen M, Kawahara H, Kawahara Y, Westerink BH (1997) The locus coeruleus noradrenergic system in the rat brain studied by dual-probe microdialysis. Brain Res 763:56-62.

Van Spanning HW, van Zwieten PA (1973) The interference of tricyclic antidepressants with the central hypotensive effect of clonidine. Eur J Pharmacol 24:402-404.

Zebrowska-Lupina I (1980) Presynaptic alpha-adrenoceptors and the action of tricyclic antidepressant drugs in behavioural despair in rats. Psychopharmacology (Berl) 71:169-172.

Zubenko GS, Cohen BM, Lipinski JF Jr, Jonas JM (1984) Clonidine in the treatment of mania and mixed bipolar disorder. Am J Psychiatry 141:1617-1618.

Dop Strengtheners

Li SX, Perry KW, Wong DT (2002) Influence of fluoxetine on the ability of bupropion to modulate extracellular dopamine and norepinephrine concentrations in three mesocorticolimbic areas of rats. Neuropharmacology 42:181-190.

Zocchi A, Varnier G, Arban R, Griffante C, Zanetti L, Bettelini L, Marchi M, Gerrard PA, Corsi M (2003) Effects of antidepressant drugs and GR 205171, an neurokinin-1 (NK1) receptor antagonist, on the response in the forced swim test and on monoamine extracellular levels in the frontal cortex of the mouse. Neurosci Lett 345:73-76.

Mixed Drugs
Tricyclic Antidepressants
Brosen K (2004) Some aspects of genetic polymorphism in the biotransformation of antidepressants. Therapie 59:5-12.

Jordan S, Kramer GL, Zukas PK, Moeller M, Petty F (1994) In vivo biogenic amine efflux in medial prefrontal cortex with imipramine, fluoxetine, and fluvoxamine. Synapse 18:294-297.

Maione S, Palazzo E, Pallotta M, Leyva J, Berrino L, Rossi F (1997) Effects of imipramine on raphe nuclei and prefrontal cortex extracellular serotonin levels in the rat. Psychopharmacology (Berl) 134:401-405.

Intracellular drugs
Kovacs P, Hernadi I (2002) Iontophoresis of lithium antagonizes noradrenergic action on prefrontal neurons of the rat. Brain Res 947:150-156.

Manji HK, Hsiao JK, Risby ED, Oliver J, Rudorfer MV, Potter WZ (1991) The mechanisms of action of lithium. I. Effects on serotoninergic and noradrenergic systems in normal subjects. Arch Gen Psychiatry 48:505-512.

Chapter 10. Overt Mental Illnesses
Halliday GM (2001) A review of the neuropathology of schizophrenia. Clin Exp Pharmacol Physiol 28:64-65.

Depression
Asnis GM, McGinn LK, Sanderson WC (1995) Atypical depression: clinical aspects and noradrenergic function. Am J Psychiatry 152:31-36.

Brody AL, Saxena S, Fairbanks LA, Alborzian S, Demaree HA,

Maidment KM, Baxter LR Jr. (2000) Personality changes in adult subjects with major depressive disorder or obsessive-compulsive disorder treated with paroxetine. J Clin Psychiatry 61:349-355.

Correa H, Duval F, Claude MM, Bailey P, Tremeau F, Diep TS, Crocq MA, Castro JO, Macher JP (2001) Noradrenergic dysfunction and antidepressant treatment response. Eur Neuropsychopharmacol 11:163-168.

Joyce PR, Mulder RT, McKenzie JM, Luty SE, Cloninger CR (2004) Atypical depression, atypical temperament and a differential anti-depressant response to fluoxetine and nortriptyline. Depress Anxiety 19:180-186.

John J Ratey, Catherine Johnson, *Shadow Syndromes*, Bantam Books, New York, NY, 1998, p.82 (quote of Dr. Mark George).

Roy A, Pickar D, Linnoila M, Potter WZ (1985) Plasma norepinephrine level in affective disorders. Relationship to melancholia. Arch Gen Psychiatry 42:1181-1185.

Salomon RM, Miller HL, Delgado PL, Charney D (1993) The use of tryptophan depletion to evaluate central serotonin function in depression and other neuropsychiatric disorders. Int Clin Psychopharmacol Nov;8 Suppl 2:41-6.

Scatton B, Loo H, Dennis T, Benkelfat C, Gay C, Poirier-Littre MF (1986) Decrease in plasma levels of 3,4-dihydroxyphenylethyleneglycol in major depression. Psychopharmacology (Berl) 88:220-225.

Bipolar Disorder

Samuel H Barondes, *Molecules and Mental Illness*, Scientific American

Library, New York, NY, 1993.

Horrigan JP, Barnhill LJ (1999) Guanfacine and secondary mania in children. J Affect Disord 54:309-314.

Jimerson DC, Nurnberger JI Jr, Post RM, Gershon ES, Kopin IJ (1981) Plasma MHPG in rapid cyclers and healthy twins. Arch Gen Psychiatry 38:1287-1290.

Joyce PR, Fergusson DM, Woollard G, Abbott RM, Horwood LJ, Upton J (1995) Urinary catecholamines and plasma hormones predict mood state in rapid cycling bipolar affective disorder. J Affect Disorder 33:233-243.

Ostrow D, Halaris A, Dysken M, DeMet E, Harrow M, Davis J (1984) State dependence of noradrenergic activity in a rapid cycling bipolar patient. J Clin Psychiatry 45:306-309.

Unnerstall JR, Fernandez I, Orensanz LM (1985) The alpha-adrenergic receptor: radiohistochemical analysis of functional characteristics and biochemical differences. Pharmacol Biochem Behav 22:859-874.

Seasonal Affective Disorder (SAD)

Avery DH, Eder DN, Bolte MA, Hellekson CJ, Dunner DL, Vitiello MV, Prinz PN (2001) Dawn simulation and bright light in the treatment of SAD: a controlled study. Biol Psychiatry 50:205-216.

Goel N, Terman M, Terman JS (2003) Dimensions of temperament and bright light response in seasonal affective disorder. Psychiatry Res 119:89-97.

Rudorfer MV, Skwerer RG, Rosenthal NE (1993) Biogenic amines in seasonal affective disorder: effects of light therapy. Psychiatry Res 46:19-28.

Schizophrenia

Caroli F, Baldacci-Epinette C, Ribeyre P (1993) Antidepressant treatment of schizophrenic patients. Encephale 19 Spec No 2:393-396.

Dina C, Nemanov L, Gritsenko I, Rosolio N, Osher Y, Heresco-Levy U, Sariashvilli E, Bachner-Melman R, Zohar AH, Benjamin J, Belmaker RH, Ebstein RP (2004) Fine mapping of a region on chromosome 8p gives evidence for a QTL contributing to individual differences in an anxiety-related personality trait: TPQ harm avoidance. Am J Med Genet B Neuropsychiatr Genet 132B:104-108.

Eccleston D, Fairbairn AF, Hassanyeh F, McClelland HA, Stephens DA (1985) The effect of propranolol and thioridazine on positive and negative symptoms of schizophrenia. Br J Psychiatry 147:623-630.

Freedman R, Kirch D, Bell J, Adler LE, Pecevich M, Pachtman E, Denver P (1982) Clonidine treatment of schizophrenia. Double-blind comparison to placebo and neuroleptic drugs. Acta Psychiatr Scand 65:35-45.

Garver DL, Steinberg JL, McDermott BE, Yao JK, Ramberg JE, Lewis S, Kingsbury SJ (1997) Etiologic heterogeneity of the psychoses: is there a dopamine psychosis? Neuropsychopharmacol 16:191-201.

Goff DC, Brotman AW, Waites M, McCormick S (1990) Trial of fluoxetine added to neuroleptics for treatment-resistant schizophrenic patients. Am J Psychiatry 147:492-494.

Golimbet VE, Alfimova MV, Manandian KK, Abramova LI, Kaleda VG, Mitiushina NG, Oleichik IV, Iurov IuB, Trubnikov VI (2001) Serotonin type 2a (5-HTR2A) receptor gene polymorphism and personality traits in patients with endogenous psychoses. Genetika 37:545-548.

Kramer MS, Vogel WH, DiJohnson C, Dewey DA, Sheves P, Cavicchia S, Little P, Schmidt R, Kimes I (1989) Antidepressants in 'depressed' schizophrenic inpatients. A controlled trial. Arch Gen Psychiatry 46:922-928.

Lieberman J, Jody D, Geisler S, Alvir J, Loebel A, Szymanski S, Woerner M, Borenstein M (1993) Time course and biologic correlates of treatment response in first-episode schizophrenia. Arch Gen Psychiatry 50:369-376.

Maas JW, Miller AL, Tekell JL, Funderburg L, Silva JA, True J, Velligan D, Berman N, Bowden CL (1995) Clonidine plus haloperidol in the treatment of schizophrenia/psychosis. J Clin Psychopharmacol 15:361-364.

Poyurovsky M, Hermesh H, Weizman A (1996) Fluvoxamine treatment in clozapine-induced obsessive-compulsive symptoms in schizophrenic patients. Clin Neuropharmacol 19:305-313.

Poyurovsky M, Isakov V, Hromnikov S, Modai I, Rauchberger B, Schneidman M, Weizman A (1999) Fluvoxamine treatment of obsessive-compulsive symptoms in schizophrenic patients: an add-on open study. Int Clin Psychopharmacol 14:95-100.

Reznik I, Sirota P (2000) Obsessive and compulsive symptoms in schizophrenia: a randomized controlled trial with fluvoxamine and neuroleptics. J Clin Psychopharmacol 20:410-416.

Sayeed Khan MN, Arshad N, Ullah N (2004) Treatment outcome of schizophrenia co-morbid with obsessive-compulsive disorder. J Coll

Physicians Surg Pak 14:234-236.

Sethi BB, Dube S (1983) Propranolol in schizophrenia. Prog Neuropsychopharmacol Biol Psychiatry 7:89-99.

Sievers M, Sato T, Moller HJ, Bottlender R (2005) Obsessive-compulsive disorder (OCD) with psychotic symptoms and response to treatment with SRI. Pharmacopsychiatry 38:104-105.

Solomon H Snyder, *Madness and the Brain*, McGraw-Hill, New York, NY, 1975.

Stockmeier CA, DiCarlo JJ, Zhang Y, Thompson P, Meltzer HY (1993) Characterization of typical and atypical antipsychotic drugs based on in vivo occupancy of serotonin2 and dopamine2 receptors. J Pharmacol Exp Ther 266:1374-1384.

Thakore JH, Berti C, Dinan TG (1996) An open trial of adjunctive sertraline in the treatment of chronic schizophrenia. Acta Psychiatr Scand 94:194-197.

Van Kammen DP, Peter JL, van Kammen WB, Rosen J, Yao JK, McAdam D, Linnoila M (1989) Clonidine treatment of schizophrenia: can we predict treatment response? Psychiatry Res 27:297-311.

Yamamoto K, Hornykiewicz O (2004) Proposal for a noradrenaline hypothesis of schizophrenia. Prog Neuropsychopharmacol Biol Psychiatry 28:913-922.

Attention Deficit Hyperactivity Disorder (ADHD)

J Raymond DePaulo, Leslie Alan Horvitz, *Understanding Depression*, Wiley, Hoboken, NJ, 2002, pp. 61-63.

Gaffney GR, Perry PJ, Lund BC, Bever-Stille KA, Arndt S, Kuperman S (2002) Risperidone versus clonidine in the treatment of children and adolescents with Tourette's syndrome. J Am Acad Child Adolesc Psychiatry 41:330-336.

George Isaac, *Bipolar not ADHD*, Writers Club Press, Lincoln, Nebraska, 2001.

Jimenez-Jimenez FJ, Garcia-Ruiz PJ (2001) Pharmacological options for the treatment of Tourette's disorder. Drugs 61:2207-2220.

Robertson M (2006) Attention deficit hyperactivity disorder, tics and Tourette's syndrome: the relationship and treatment implications. A commentary. Eur Child Adolesc Psychiatry 15:1-11.

Spencer T, Biederman J, Wilens T, Steingard R, Geist D (1993) Nortriptyline treatment of children with attention-deficit hyperactivity disorder and tic disorder or Tourette's syndrome. J Am Acad Child Adolesc Psychiatry 32:205-210.

Anxiety

Kathol RG, Noyes R, Slymen DJ, Crowe RR, Clancy J, Kerber RE (1980) Propranolol in chronic anxiety disorders. A controlled study. Arch Gen Psychiatry. 37:1361-1365.

Meibach RC, Dunner D, Wilson LG, Ishiki D, Dager SR (1987) Comparative efficacy of propranolol, chlordiazepoxide, and placebo in the treatment of anxiety: a double-blind trial. J Clin Psychiatry 48:355-358.

Peet M, Ali S (1986) Propranolol and atenolol in the treatment of anxiety. Int Clin Psychopharmacol 1:314-319.

Rossi S, Singer S, Shearman E, Sershen H, Lajtha A (2005) The effects of cholinergic and dopaminergic antagonists on nicotine-induced cerebral neurotransmitter changes. Neurchem Res 30: 541-558.

Sanger DJ (1988) Behavioural effects of the alpha 2-adrenoceptor antagonists idazoxan and yohimbine in rats: comparisons with amphetamine. Psychopharmacol (Berl) 96:243-249.

Singer S, Rossi S, Verzosa S, Hashim A, Lonow R, Cooper T, Sershen H, Lajtha A (2004) Nicotine-induced changes in neurotransmitter levels in brain areas associated with cognitive function. Neurochem Res 29: 1779-1792.

Soderpalm A, Blomqvist O, Soderpalm B (1995) The yohimbine-induced anticonflict effect in the rat, Part I. Involvement of noradrenergic, serotonergic and endozepinergic(?) mechanisms. J Neural Transm Gen Sect 100:175-189.

Drug and Alcohol Abuse
Andreas K, Fischer HD, Schimdt J (1983) [Effect of central effective substances on alcohol preference.] Biomed Biochim Acta 42:391-398.

Le AD, Harding S, Juzytsch W, Funk D, Shaham Y (2005) Role of alpha-2 adrenoceptors in stress-induced reinstatement of alcohol seeking and alcohol self-administration in rats. Psychopharmacology (Berl) 179:366-373.

Personality Disorders
Paris J, Zweig-Frank H, Kin NM, Schwartz G, Steiger H, Nair NP (2004) Neurobiological correlates of diagnosis and underlying traits in patients with borderline personality disorder compared with normal controls. Psychiatry Res 121:239-252.

Impulse Control Disorders

Campbell M, Gonzalez NM, Silva RR (1992) The pharmacologic treatment of conduct disorders and rage outbursts. Psychiatr Clin North Am 15:69-85.

Mattes JA (1986) Psychopharmacology of temper outbursts. A review. J Nerv Ment Dis 174:464-470.

Eating Disorders

Simpson SG, al-Mufti R, Andersen AE, DePaul JR (1992) Bipolar II affective disorder in eating disorder inpatients. J Nerv Ment Dis 180:719-722.

Chapter 11. Expanded Dysthymia

Peter D Kramer, *Listening to Prozac*, Viking Penguin, New York, NY, 1993, p.197.

John J Ratey, Catherine Johnson, *Shadow Syndromes*, Bantam Books, New York, NY, 1998, p.11.

Chapter 12. Personality
Cloninger's Big Three Model

Cloninger CR (1986) A unified biosocial theory of personality and its role in the development of anxiety states. Psychiatr Develop 3:167-226.

Cloninger CR (1987) A systematic method for clinical description and classification of personality variants: a proposal. Arch Gen Psych 44:573-588.

De Saint Hilaire Z, Straub J, Pelissolo A (2005) Temperament and character in primary insomnia. Eur Psychiatry 20:188-192.

Gerra G, Zaimovic A, Timpano M, Zambelli U, Delsignore R, Brambilla F (2000) Neuroendocrine correlates of temperamental traits in humans. Psychoneuroendocrinology 25:479-496.

Gutierrez-Zotes JA, Bayon C, Montserrat C, Valero J, Labad A, Cloninger CR, Fernandez-Aranda F (2004) Temperament and Character Inventory Revised (TCI-R). Standardization and normative data in a general population sample. Actas Esp Psiquiatr 32:8-15.

Hennig J, Toll C, Schonlau P, Rohrmann S, Netter P (2000) Endocrine responses after d-fenfluramine and ipsapirone challenge: further support for Cloninger's tridimensional model of personality. Neuropsychobiology 41:38-47.

Mitropoulou V, Trestman RL, New AS, Flory JD, Silverman JM, Siever LJ (2003) Neurobiologic function and temperament in subjects with personality disorders. CNS Spectr 8:725-730.

Peirson AR, Heuchert JW, Thomala L, Berk M, Plein H, Cloninger CR (1999) Relationship between serotonin and the temperament and character inventory. Psychiatry Res 89:29-37.

Swann AC, Johnson BA, Cloninger CR, Chen YR (1999) Relationships of plasma tryptophan availability to course of illness and clinical features of alcoholism: a preliminary study. Psychopharmacology (Berl) 143:380-384.

Weijers HG, Wiesbeck GA, Jakob F, Boning J (2001) Neuroendocrine responses to fenfluramine and its relationship to personality in alcoholism. J Neural Transm 108:1093-1105.

The Enneagram Model

Don Richard Riso, Russ Hudson, *Personality Types: Using the Enneagram for Self-Discovery*, Houghton Mifflin, New York, NY, 1996.

Chapter 13. Dominance and Leadership

Baenninger R (1968) Catechol amines and social relations in Siamese fighting fish. Anim Behav 16:442-447.

Higley JD, Suomi SJ, Linnoila M (1996) A nonhuman primate model of type II alcoholism? Part 2. Diminished social competence and excessive aggression correlates with low cerebrospinal fluid 5-hydroxyindoleacetic acid concentrations. Alcohol Clin Exp Res 20:643-650.

Kaplan JR, Manuck SB, Fontenot MB, Mann JJ (2002) Central nervous system monoamine correlates of social dominance in cynomolgus monkeys (Macaca fascicularis). Neuropsychopharmacol 26:431-443.

Lawrence CW, Haynes JR (1970) Epinephrine and nore-epinephrine effects on social dominance behavior. Psychol Rep 27:195-198.

Malatynska E, Kostowski W (1984) The effect of antidepressant drugs on dominance behavior in rats competing for food. Pol J Pharmacol Pharm 36:531-540.

Redmond DE, Maas JW, Kling A, Dekirmenjian H (1971) Changes in primate social behavior after treatment with alpha-methyl-para-tyrosine. Psychosom Med 33:97-113.

Chapter 14. Evolution

J Raymond DePaulo, Leslie Alan Horvitz, *Understanding Depression*, Wiley, Hoboken, NJ, 2002, pp.254-258.

Jared Diamond, *Guns, Germs, and Steel: The Fates of Human Societies*, Norton, New York, NY, 1999.

Chapter 15. Genetics

Bobb et al. (2005) Support for association between ADHD and two candidate genes: NET1 and DRD1. Am J Med Genet B Neuropsychiatr Genet 134:67-72.

Fan JB, Sklar P (2005) Meta-analysis reveals association between serotonin transporter gene STin2 VNTR polymorphism and schizophrenia. Mol Psychiatry 10:928-938.

Inoue K, Itoh K, Yoshida K, Shimizu T, Suzuki T (2004) Positive association between T-182C polymorphism in the norepinephrine transporter gene and susceptibility to major depressive disorder in a japanese population. Neuropsychobiology 50:301-304.

Lotrich FE, Pollock BG, Ferrell RE (2001) Polymorphism of the serotonin transporter: implications for the use of selective serotonin reuptake inhibitors. Am J Pharmacogenomics 1:153-164.

Norton N, Owen MJ (2005) HTR2A: association and expression studies in neuropsychiatric genetics. Ann Med 37:121-129.

Ueno S (2003) Genetic polymorphisms of serotonin and dopamine transporters in mental disorders. J Med Invest 50:25-31.

Chapter 16. The Role of Talk Therapy

Aaron T. Beck, *Cognitive Therapy and the Emotional Disorders*, Plume, New York, NY, 1979.

Brody et al. (2001) Regional brain metabolic changes in patients with major depression treated with either paroxetine or interpersonal therapy: preliminary findings. Arch Gen Psychiatry 58:631-640.

Viktor E Frankl, *Man's Search for Meaning: An Introduction to Logotherapy*, Beacon Press, Boston, MA, 1959.

Furmark T, Tillfors M, Marteinsdottir I, Fischer H, Pissiota A, Langstron B, Fredrikson M (2002) Common changes in cerebral blood flow in patients with social phobia treated with citalopram or cognitive-behavioral therapy. Arch Gen Psychiatry 59:425-433.

Goldapple K, Segal Z, Garson C, Lau M, Bieling P, Kennedy S, Mayberg H (2004) Modulation of cortical-limbic pathways in major depression: treatment-specific effects of cognitive behavior therapy. Arch Gen Psychiatry 61:34-41.

Martin SD, Martin E, Rai SS, Richardson MA, Royall R (2001) Brain blood flow changes in depressed patients treated with interpersonal psychotherapy or venlafaxine hydrochloride: preliminary findings. Arch Gen Psychiatry 58:641-648.

Stephen A Mitchell, Margaret J Black, *Freud and Beyond: A History of Modern Psychoanalytic Thought*, Basic Books, New York, NY, 1995.

Prasko et al. (2004) The change of regional brain metabolism (18FDG PET) in panic disorder during the treatment with cognitive behavioral therapy or antidepressants. Neuro Endocrinol Lett 25:340-348.

Roffman JL, Marci CD, Glick DM, Dougherty DD, Rauch SL (2005) Neuroimaging and the functional neuroanatomy of psychotherapy. Psychol Med 35:1385-1398.

Carl Rogers, *On Becoming a Person: A Therapist's View of Psychotherapy*, Houghton Mifflin, New York, NY, 1961.

BF Skinner, *About Behaviorism*, Vintage, New York, NY, 1974.

Straube T, Glauer M, Dilger S, Mentzel HJ, Miltner WH (2006) Effects of cognitive-behavioral therapy on brain activation in specific phobia. Neuroimage 29:125-135.

Wykes T, Brammer M, Mellers J, Bray P, Reeder C, Williams C, Corner J (2002) Effects on the brain of a psychological treatment: cognitive remediation therapy: functional magnetic resonance imaging in schizophrenia. Br J Psychiatry 181:144-152.

Chapter 17. New Directions for Improving Psychiatry

Abiodun OA (2005) Role of radiology in psychiatry: a review. East Afr Med J 82:260-266.

Chugani DC, Chugani HT (2000) PET: mapping of serotonin synthesis. Adv Neurol 83:165-171.

Chugani DC, Muzik O (2000) Alpha[C-11]methyl-L-tryptophan PET maps brain serotonin synthesis and kynurenine pathway metabolism. J Cereb Blood Flow Metab 20:2-9.

Chugani DC, Muzik O, Chakraborty P, Mangner T, Chugani HT (1998) Human brain serotonin synthesis capacity measured in vivo with alpha-[C-11]methyl-L-tryptophan. Synapse 28:33-43.

Chugani DC, Niimura K, Chaturvedi S, Muzik O, Fakhouri M, Lee ML, Chugani HT (1999) Increased brain serotonin synthesis in migraine. Neurology 53:1473-1479.

Dhaenen H (2001) Imaging the serotonergic system in depression. Eur Arch Psychiatry Clin Neurosci 251 Suppl 2:II76-80.

Fu X, Tan PZ, Kula NS, Baldessarini R, Tamagnan G, Innis RB, Baldwin RM (2002) Synthesis, receptor potency, and selectivity of halogenated diphenylpiperidines as serotonin 5-HT2A ligands for PET or SPECT brain imaging. J Med Chem 45:2319-2324.

Hagberg GE, Torstenson R, Marteinsdottir I, Fredrikson M, Langstrom B, Blomqvist G (2002) Kinetic compartment modeling of [11C]-5-hydroxy-L-tryptophan for positron emission tomography assessment of serotonin synthesis in human brain. J Cereb Blood Flow Metab 22:1352-1366.

Laakso A, Hietala J (2000) PET studies of brain monoamine transporters. Curr Pharm Des 6:1611-1623.

Lundkvist C, Halldin C, Ginovart N, Nyberg S, Swahn CG, Carr AA, Brunner F, Farde L (1996) [11C]MDL 100907, a radioligland for selective imaging of 5-HT(2A) receptors with positron emission tomography. Life Sci 58:PL 187-192.

Nakai A, Diksic M, Kumakura Y, D'Souza D, Kersey K (2005) The effects of the 5-HT3 antagonist, alosetron, on brain serotonin synthesis in patients with irritable bowel syndrome. Neurogastroenterol Motil 17:212-221.

Shoaf SE, Carson R, Hommer D, Williams W, Higley JD, Schmall B, Herscovitch P, Eckelman W, Linnoila M (1998) Brain serotonin synthesis rates in rhesus monkeys determined by [11C]alpha-methyl-L-tryptophan and positron emission tomography compared to CSF 5-hydroxyindole-3-acetic acid concentrations. Neuropsychopharmacology 19:345-353.

Smith KA, Morris JS, Friston KJ, Cowen PJ, Dolan RJ (1999) Brain mechanisms associated with depressive relapse and associated cognitive impairment following acute tryptophan depletion. Br J Psychiatry 174:525-529.

Sobrio F, Amokhtari M, Gourand F, Dhilly M, Dauphin F, Barre L (2000) Radiosynthesis of [18F]Lu29-024: a potential PET ligand for brain imaging of the serotonergic 5-HT2 receptor. Bioorg Med Chem 8:2511-2518.

Young SN, Leyton M, Benkelfat C (1999) Pet studies of serotonin synthesis in the human brain. Adv Exp Med Biol 467:11-18.

Improving the Current Theory

Chez MG, Aimonovitch M, Buchanan T, Mrazek S, Tremb RJ (2004) Treating autistic spectrum disorders in children: utility of the cholinesterase inhibitor rivastigmine tartrate. J Child Neurol 19:165-169.

Gross HA, Dunner DL, Lafleur D, Meltzer HL, Muhlbauder HL, Fieve RR (1977) Prostaglandins. A review of neurophysiology and psychiatric implications. Arch Gen Psychiatry 34:1189-1196.

Hong CJ, Lai IC, Liou LL, Tsai SJ (2004) Association study of the human partially duplicated alpha7 nicotinic acetylcholine receptor genetic variant with bipolar disorder. Neurosci Lett 355:6972.

Leiva DB (1990) The neurochemistry of mania: a hypothesis of etiology and rationale for treatment. Prog Neuropsychopharmacol Biol Psychiatry 14:423-429.

Paul IA, Skolnick P (2003) Glutamate and depression: clinical and preclinical studies. Ann N Y Acad Sci 1003:250-272.

Petty F, Trivedi MH, Fulton M, Rush AJ (1995) Benzodiazepines as antidepressants: does GABA play a role in depression? Biol Psychiatry 38:578-591.

Singh A, Potter A, Newhouse P (2004) Nicotinic acetylcholine receptor system and neuropsychiatric disorders. IDrugs 7:1096-1103.

Wang et al. (2004) Evidence of common and specific genetic effects: association of the muscarinic acetylcholine receptor M2 (CHRM2) gene with alcohol dependence and major depressive syndrome. Hum Mol Genet 13:1903-1911.

Zarate CA, Payne JL, Quiroz J, Sporn J, Denicoff KK, Luckenbaugh D, Charney DS, Manji HK (2004) An open-label trial of riluzole in patients with treatment-resistant major depression. Am J Psychiatry 161:171-174.

Zarate CA, Quiroz JA, Singh JB, Denicoff KD, DeJesus G, Luckenbaugh DA, Charney DS, Manji HK (2005) An open-label trial of the glutamate-modulating agent riluzole in combination with lithium for the treatment of bipolar depression. Biol Psychiatry 57:430-432.

Using Existing Drugs More Effectively
Keller S, Frishman WH (2003) Neuropsychiatric effects of cardiovascular drug therapy. Cardiol Rev 11:73-93.

Creating New Drugs
Mattson RJ, Catt JD, Sloan CP, Gao Q, Carter RB, Gentile A, Mahle CD, Matos FF, McGovern R, VanderMaelen CP, Yocca FD (2003) Development of a presynaptic 5-HT1A antagonist. Bioorg Med Chem Lett 13:285-288.

The Drug Companies

Marcia Angell, *The Truth About the Drug Companies: How They Deceive Us and What to Do About It*, Random House, New York, NY, 2004.

Merrill Goozner, *The $800 Million Pill: The Truth Behind the Cost of New Drugs*, University of California Press, Berkeley, CA, 2004.

Chapter 18. Closing Thoughts

Aldous Huxley, *Brave New World*, Harper & Brothers, New York, NY, 1932.

General References

American Psychiatric Association: *Diagnostic and Statistical Manual of Mental Disorders*, Fourth Edition, Text Revision; American Psychiatric Association, Washington, DC, 2000.

Samuel H Barondes, *Better than Prozac*, Oxford Univ Press, New York, NY, 2003.

Avery Z Conner, *Fevers of the Mind*, PublishAmerica, Frederick, Maryland, 2002.

Avery Z Conner, *100 Questions Psychiatry Should Face*, iUniverse, Lincoln, Nebraska, 2002.

Frederick K Goodwin, Kay R Jamison, *Manic-Depressive Illness*, Oxford Univ Press, New York, NY, 1990.

Kay R Jamison, *An Unquiet Mind*, Knopf, New York, NY, 1995.

Kay R Jamison, *Touched with Fire*, Free Press, New York, NY, 1993.

Eric R Kandel, James H Schwartz, Thomas M Jessell, *Principles of Neural Science, 4th Edition*, McGraw-Hill Medical, New York, NY, 2000. Peter D Kramer, *Against Depression*, Viking Penguin, New York, NY, 2005.

Peter D Kramer, *Listening to Prozac*, Viking Penguin, New York, NY, 1993.

Paul R McHugh, Phillip R Slavney, *The Perspectives of Psychiatry, 2nd Edition*, The Johns Hopkins University Press, Baltimore, MD, 1998.

John Nolte, *The Human Brain*, Mosby-Year Book, St. Louis, Missouri, 1993.

Michael J Norden, *Beyond Prozac*, ReganBooks, New York, NY, 1995.

SUMMARY OF DRUGS

Ser strengtheners

Ser reuptake inhibitors (SRIs)

Prozac (fluoxetine)

Zoloft (sertraline)

Paxil (paroxetine)

Lexapro (citalopram)

Luvox (fluvoxamine)

Ser weakeners

Atypical antipsychotics

Clozaril (clozapine)

Zyprexa (olanzapine)

Seroquel (quetiapine)

Risperdal (risperidone)

Geodon (ziprasidone)

Typical antipsychotics (see Dop weakeners)

Ser reuptake enhancers

tianeptine—not available in the United States

5HT_2A blockers

cyproheptadine

Serzone (nefazodone)

Desyrel (trazodone)

mianserin

ketanserin

Hallucinogens

LSD—lysergic acid diethylamide

Nore strengtheners

Nore reuptake inhibitors (NRIs)
> Norpramin (desipramine)
> Pamelor (nortriptyline)
> Vivactil (protriptyline)
> Strattera (atomoxetine)
> reboxetine—available in Europe

Nore weakeners

Alpha 2 adrenergic agonists
> Catapres (clonidine)
> Tenex (guanfacine)
> Wytensin (guanabenz acetate)
> Zanaflex (tizanidine)
> lofexidine—available in the United Kingdom

Beta blockers
> Inderal (propranolol)

Alpha blockers

Dop strengtheners

Antidepressants
> Wellbutrin (bupropion)

Stimulants
> Ritalin (methylphenidate)
> Adderall (amphetamine)
> cocaine

Dop weakeners

Atypical antipsychotics (see Ser weakeners)
Typical antipsychotics

Thorazine (chlorpromazine)

Haldol (haloperidol)

Mixed drugs

Certain tricyclic antidepressants

Elavil (amitriptyline)

Tofranil (imipramine)

MAO inhibitors

Parnate (tranylcypromine)

Other antidepressants

Cymbalta (duloxetine)

Effexor (venlafaxine)

Intracellular drugs

Mood stabilizers

lithium

Depakote (valproate)

Tegretol (carbamazepine)

*Capitalized: United States name

Lower case: generic name

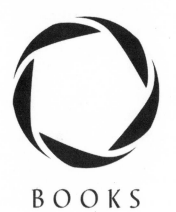

O books
O is a symbol of the world, of oneness and unity. In different cultures it also means the "eye", symbolizing knowledge and insight, and in Old English it means "place of love or home". O books explores the many paths of understanding which different traditions have developed down the ages, particularly those today that express respect for the planet and all of life.

For more information on the full list of over 300 titles please visit our website **www.O-books.net**

myspiritradio is an exciting web, internet, podcast and mobile phone global broadcast network for all those interested in teaching and learning in the fields of body, mind, spirit and self development. Listeners can hear the show online via computer or mobile phone, and even download their favourite shows to listen to on MP3 players whilst driving, working, or relaxing.

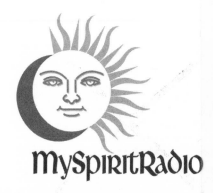

Feed your mind, change your life with O Books, The O Books radio programme carries interviews with most authors, sharing their wisdom on life, the universe and everything...e mail questions and co-create the show with O Books and myspiritradio.

Just visit **www.myspiritradio.com** for more information.